HEMORRHAGIC STROKE - AN UPDATE

Edited by **Amit Agrawal**

Hemorrhagic Stroke - An Update
http://dx.doi.org/10.5772/63253
Edited by Amit Agrawal

Contributors

Shankar Ayyappan Kutty, Sankalp Gokhale, Shazia Mirza, Alexander Khalessi, J. Scott Pannell, Arvin Wali, Kevin Porras, Peter Abraham, Michael G Brandel, David Santiago-Dieppa, Jeffrey Steinberg, Amit Agrawal, Ravi Dadlani

Published by InTech

Janeza Trdine 9, 51000 Rijeka, Croatia

Publishing Process Manager Romina Skomersic
Technical Editor SPi Global
Cover InTech Design team

First published October, 2017
Printed in Croatia
Legal deposit, Croatia: National and University Library in Zagreb

Additional hard copies can be obtained from orders@intechopen.com

Hemorrhagic Stroke - An Update, Edited by Amit Agrawal
p. cm.
Print ISBN 978-953-51-3521-0
Online ISBN 978-953-51-3522-7

Meet the editor

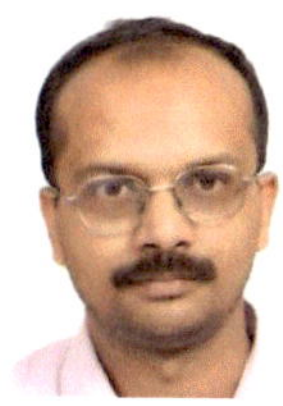

Dr. Amit Agrawal completed his neurosurgery training from the National Institute of Mental Health and Neurosciences, Bangalore, India, in the year 2003. Dr. Agrawal is a self-motivated, enthusiastic, and result-oriented professional with over 12 years of rich experience in research and development, as well as teaching and mentoring in the field of neurosurgery. He is proficient in managing and leading teams for running successful process operations and has experience of developing procedures and service standards of excellence. He has attended and participated in many international and national level symposiums and conferences and delivered lectures on vivid topics. He has published more than 500 articles in the medical field covering various topics in various national and international journals. His expertise is in identifying training needs, designing training modules, and executing the same while working with limited resources. He has excellent communication, presentation, and interpersonal skills with proven abilities in teaching and training for various academic and professional courses. Presently, he is working at the Narayana Medical College and Hospital, Nellore, AP, India.

Contents

Preface

The present book "Hemorrhagic Stroke - An Update" includes the updated information for professionals who are involved in the management of spontaneous intracerebral hemorrhage. Primary spontaneous intracerebral hemorrhage (SICH) denotes a spontaneous hemorrhage into the brain parenchyma without any secondary cause and carries a 30-day mortality of up to 50%, and causes significant and persistent disability in survivors. In the book: the authors address most difficult and challenging issues in the management and rehabilitation of SICH patients. The book one contains detail information about the pathophysiology of spontaneous intracerebral hemorrhage, neuroimaging approach in intracerebral hemorrhage, how to go about surgical intervention decision making in these patients and the rehabilitation issues in acute care and in long term survivors. I hope the collective contribution from experts will make this book to be valuable guide to further develop their understanding about spontaneous intracerebral hemorrhage. I am grateful to all of the authors who have contributes their tremendous expertise to the present book, my wife and daughter for their passionate support and last but not least I wish to acknowledge the outstanding support from Ms. Romina Skomersic, Publishing Process manger, InTech Open Science Croatia who collaborated tirelessly in crafting this book.

Amit Agrawal
Department of Neurosurgery
Narayana Medical College and Hospital
Chinthareddypalem
Nellore (AP), India

Chapter 1

Introductory Chapter: An Introduction to Hypertension-Related Intracerebral Hematomas

Ravi Dadlani and Amit Agrawal

Additional information is available at the end of the chapter

http://dx.doi.org/10.5772/intechopen.70048

1. Introduction

Of all cerebral strokes, hemorrhagic stroke forms approximately 15%, of which hypertensive intracranial hematomas (HIH) constitute the vast majority [1, 2]. Intracranial hemorrhage (ICH), contrary to popular belief, is not a 'modern disease' and is mentioned as 'Cerebral Apoplexy' in the writings of antiquity credited to Hippocrates [3]. ICH can be attributed to a number of underlying pathologies including amyloid angiopathy, cryptic vascular malformations, arteritis and hypertension [3]. Despite modern imaging such as computed tomography (CT) and magnetic resonance imaging (MRI), diagnostic uncertainty inhibits a serious study of the natural history and epidemiology of ICH [3]. ICH is predominantly of two types: primary ICH, when no underlying pathology is identifiable and secondary ICH, when hemorrhage occurs in a pre-existing lesion such as a tumor or arteriovenous malformation [2, 3].

ICH occurring spontaneously is often referred to as 'Hypertensive' in common medical parlance, and there is little doubt that elevated blood pressures promote the occurrence of ICH; although several environmental factors have been identified as risk factors, hypertension remains the single most relevant of them all [3]. A systematic review of literature has demonstrated that hypertension is one of the commonest and most prevalent risk factors associated with ICH [1, 4]. A 3.5-fold increase in the incidence of ICH is noted in hypertensive patients in comparison with normotensive patients [2]. Isolated systolic hypertension is found to correlate most strongly with ICH in contrast to diastolic hypertension and borderline isolated systolic hypertension [1]. The other factors found to have some relevance to the occurrence of ICH are cigarette smoking(increases risk of ICH by 4x to 5x), alcohol consumption, diabetes mellitus, use of oral contraceptives and male gender [1, 3]. There has also been an association between low mean serum cholesterol and the incidence of ICH, especially in the older individuals [3, 5]. HIH also has a racial predilection, being highest in Asian population and least in the Caucasians [3]. Of the myriad diseases being studied today, HIH is not only one of the many which is being investigated so thoroughly that a clear understanding of the risk factors and their modifications has attributed to the plunging incidence of the disease [3].

2. Clinical presentation

Clinical symptomatology of the ICH is dependent on the dissection of the brain tissue by the expanding hematoma and mass effect, implying the importance of the location and size of the hematoma [6]. Location of HIH is usually in the deep nuclei of the brain: basal ganglia (40%), the thalamus (10–25%), the cerebellum (5–10%) and the pons (5%) [6]. Thalamic hematomas may further be subdivided into four different locations: anterolateral (21%), medial (15%), posterolateral (55%) and dorsal (9%) [7]. Lobar hematomas involving the neocortex account for 20% or less [6]. The hallmark of ICH is 'Acute neurological deficit with rapid progression,' in contrast to ischemic strokes [6]. Fluctuating neurological symptoms are extremely uncommon [6]. The general symptoms include raised intracranial pressure which manifests as headache (33–57%), nausea and vomiting (29–46%) and decrease in the level of consciousness (28–37%)] [6]. At presentation, 4–20% of ICH patients are in a coma [6]. Meningeal irritation manifesting as neck stiffness and seizures (<10%)] are other general symptoms of ICH [6]. Symptomatology related to the location of the hematoma varies. Cortical lobar hematomas in the dominant hemisphere can present with higher mental function symptoms such as aphasia, acalculia or motor apraxia [6]. Non-dominant hemispheric symptoms appear as left-side neglect, agnosia or visuospatial dysfunction [6]. Hematomas may present with symptomatology specific to the cerebral lobe involved such as abulic-apathetic behaviors with frontal lobe involvement and contralateral homonymous hemianopsia with occipital lobe involvement [6]. The involvement of the deep grey nuclei usually depends on the location and direction of the hematoma expansion, e.g., caudate nuclei hematomas may involve the anterior limb of the internal capsule involving predominantly frontothalamic and frontopontine fibers manifesting as prominent neurobehavioral changes, in contrast to putaminal hematomas which usually involve the posterior limb of the internal capsule and may present with contralateral hemiparesis or hemiplegia [6]. Caudate and thalamic aphasias may occur in the dominant hemisphere [6]. Cerebellar hematomas may demonstrate the typical 'Cerebellar Syndrome,' and pontine hematomas may present with dense quadriplegia or the typical 'locked-in syndrome' in addition to cranial nerve deficits [6].

2.1. Expansion of ICH

Expansion of ICH appears to be more common than initially thought. Over a third of patients may demonstrate the expansion of hematoma over the first 24 h [6]. A fivefold morbidity has been reported with the expansion of the ICH and a significant cause of death in these patients [8]. The radiographic criteria for hematoma expansion have been reported as an increase in hematoma volume by ≥12.5 cm or by ≥1.4 times [8]. Temporally, the highest probability of hematoma expansion is seen in the hyperacute stage (17% within the first 6 h) [8]. Hematoma enlargement after 24 h rarely occurs [8]. It stands to reason, therefore, if a hyperacute CT scans reveal an ICH, repeat scans should be considered periodically. There have been speculations about the etiology of the expansion, viz. whether there occur repeated small hemorrhages or there is a continuous oozing [9]. Expansion of an ICH generally follows the general 'rule of thumb,' and the larger the hematoma at presentation, the more likely it is to expand [10].

Interestingly, hematoma expansion has been shown to be an independent determinant of morbidity and mortality in ICH [11]. For an increase of 10% in the size of the ICH, there appears to be a 5% increased hazard of death [12].

3. Pathophysiology and etiopathogenesis of ICH

It has been proven that ICH usually occurs in the area supplied by small perforating arterioles (50–700 μm in dia.) and the rupture occurs as a consequence of hypertension-related pathological changes which include fibrinoid necrosis, microaneurysm formation and lipohyalinosis [6]. It is conjectural that the pulse pressure may in fact be more important than the absolute blood pressure, since the turbulence generated would damage the vessel resulting in a rupture if collagen is inadequate especially in the presence of repetitive cycles of arteriolar dilatation [7]. The Charcôt-Bouchard aneurysm, which has been a controversy since its original description, is a fusiform dilatation of the thinning, vasculopathic arteriolar wall which virtually entirely consists of collagen [7]. The controversy has stemmed from the use of the term 'aneurysm' for the 'non-saccular,' 'fusiform' dilatation of the vessel walls [7]. These, then, morphologically, characterize a segmental disease, fusiform (dilatation by a factor of two or three, over lengths of 100–200 μm), which has been revealed by the use of alkaline phosphatase techniques and may be visualized in the pathological specimen of the hematoma as extensions of a vessel into an acute hematoma lined by a endothelial lining [7].

4. Management

The management is symptomatic and mainly supportive, and no definite treatment modality has proven to improve outcomes in ICH [6]. Mortality is high, generally ranging from 30 to 55% with a very high case fatality rate in the first 7 days [6]. The long-term prognosis for the survivors is not very encouraging with less than 30% of patients being independent at 3 months of the ICH ictus [6]. The goals of management therefore include prevention of further brain injury by deterring hematoma expansion, restricting edema and to attempt recruiting the brain's plasticity to improve the rehabilitation outcome [9]. Prehospital management is vital and primarily consists of ventilator and cardiovascular support and transporting the patient to the nearest available stroke unit [9, 13]. Management at the emergency room (ER) consists of a thorough neurological assessment, management of elevated blood pressures and neuroradiological evaluation and may entail emergency procedures such as insertion of an external ventricular drain, monitoring ICP and its management and reversal of coagulopathy [13]. Critical pathways should be formulated and followed at the

ER level [13]. Computed tomography and magnetic resonance imaging are both reasonable initial modalities of investigation, especially if the differentiation between infarction and hemorrhage is difficult clinically [13]. However, CT is considered the gold standard for the diagnosis of hemorrhage [13]. Intensive blood pressure lowering has been evaluated by several trials, and the majority of results reflect a proclivity toward rapid reduction to less than 140 mm Hg [10]. This seems clinically reasonable, generally well tolerated and appears to impact hematoma expansion in ICH [10].

4.1. Ultra-early hemostatic therapy for ICH

Ultra-early hemostatic therapy for ICH is recommended because an increase in the hematoma volume and expansion are associated with poorer outcome [12]. ICH has an increased incidence in patients on oral anticoagulants or antiplatelet drugs and those with coagulation factor deficiencies and platelet abnormalities [12]. Ultra-early hemostatic therapy is particularly indicated in these patients and includes appropriate intervention, such as platelet transfusions or administration of vitamin K, in addition to the other management options outlined above [12].

4.2. Surgical management

Early studies had failed to demonstrate any significant difference between conservative and surgical management of ICH [9]. There were also reports of poorer surgical outcome due to the trauma of surgery itself and a higher postoperative re-hemorrhage rate [7]. There have been over a dozen randomized controlled trials, addressing the issue of the surgical management of ICH [9]. The surgical approach to the hematoma depends on the location and the depth of the hematoma and eloquence of the brain involved among other considerations [9]. It has also been reported that surgery may be beneficial only if undertaken within 8 h of ictus, thus limiting the toxic effects of the blood components on the brain [14].

4.3. Recent advances and trials

The initial Surgical Trial in ICH (STICH) trial of over 1000 patients did not reveal any statistically significant benefit of surgery for supratentorial ICH except for hemorrhage within 1 cm of cortical surface [7]. The STICH II trial for lobar hematomas found a small (3.7%) absolute benefit in the surgical group, but it was riddled with controversy because of the inclusion of patients with a normal level of consciousness (i.e., clinically no evidence of raised ICP) [14]. The STICH II trial, however, did demonstrate significant benefit from surgery in the group that was considered a poor prognosis group (i.e., low GCS and a large hematoma volume) [14]. There have been several recent trials researching minimally invasive surgical techniques such as endoscopic or stereotactic aspiration with or without fibrinolytic agents [9]. 'Minimally Invasive Surgery and rtPA for Intracerebral Hemorrhage Evacuation' (MISTIE) is a series of clinical trials where minimally invasive evacuation of ICH and the use of either a thrombolytic agent [MISTIE II (2013) and MISTIE III (ongoing)] or a CT-guided endoscope (MISTIE-ICES) is under study [15]. Early results were favorable for the successful and early removal of the ICH in addition to demonstrating a fall in the mortality rate and long-term qualitative outcome [15].

4.4. Recombinant activated factor VII (rFVIIa) therapy

Recombinant activated factor VII (rFVIIa) therapy, although a well-documented therapy in the Haemophilias, it has found limited application in the indiscriminate use in ICH and is associated with multiple thromboembolic complicationsincluding death [11]. It has, however, demonstrated a reduction in the growth of the ICH when administered within 4 h of the ictus. Perihematomal edema and secondary injury are the focus of attention and includes altering events at the molecular level, which would precipitate secondary injury in ICHs. These include iron-mediated toxicity and acute inflammation which is induced by the degradation products of hemoglobin [10]. Multiple modalities, such as the use of minocycline, hypothermia and albumin, have been advocated as possible neuroprotective agents in the prevention of secondary injury from inflammation in ICH [10]. Deferoxamine mesylate is investigated to counter the neurotoxic effects of iron resulting from hemolysis of the red blood cells [10]. Preclinical work with Pioglitazone has revealed that the transcription factor peroxisome proliferator-activated receptor gamma plays an essential role in enhancing phagocytosis with the dual role of restraining oxidative stress and inflammation [10].

5. Prognosis

There is a slightly more than 1% chance of a survivor of an ICH to endure either a new ICH or an ischemic stroke each year [9]. The three most important and reliable indicators of poor outcome after ICH are volume of the hematoma, level of consciousness and intraventricular hemorrhage (IVH), which is implicated most likely due to the involvement of more centrally located structures within the brain [9, 12].

6. Conclusion

Although, hemorrhagic stroke has been known since antiquity, it has been an extremely challenging medical condition to treat. One that has been investigated exhaustively, and future avenues of treatment will most likely combine several approaches not just at reducing the size of the hematoma and prevention of its expansion but also therapies aimed at mitigating the secondary insult. Further focus, understandably, would rest on grasping the molecular mechanisms of the pathogenesis and the innate immune responses and formulating remedies to combat these effects. This chapter has attempted a brief overview of the topic. Further sections will highlight many aspects of this neurological entity in depth, hopefully illuminating our understanding of this ubiquitous but challenging disorder.

Author details

Ravi Dadlani[1*] and Amit Agrawal[2]

*Address all correspondence to: ravi.dadlani@gmail.com

1 Department of Neurosurgery, Apollo Specialty Hospitals, Nellore, Andhra Pradesh, India

2 Department of Neurosurgery, Narayna Medical College Hospital, Chinthareddypalem, Nellore, Andhra Pradesh, India

References

[1] Sessa M. Intracerebral hemorrhage and hypertension. Neurological Sciences. 2008; **29**(S2):258-259

[2] Ikram M, Wieberdink R, Koudstaal P. International epidemiology of intracerebral hemorrhage. Current Atherosclerosis Reports. 2012;**14**(4):300-306

[3] Kase C, Caplan L. Intracerebral Hemorrhage. Boston: Butterworth-Heinemann; 1994

[4] Ciccone A, Pozzi M, Motto C, Tiraboschi P, Sterzi R. Epidemiological, clinical, and therapeutic aspects of primary intracerebral hemorrhage. Neurological Sciences. 2008;**29**(S2):256-257

[5] Valappil A, Chaudhary N, Girija A, Gopalakrishnan B, Praveenkumar R. Low cholesterol as a risk factor for primary intracerebral hemorrhage: A case-control study. Annals of Indian Academy of Neurology. 2012;**15**(1):19

[6] Ko S, Choi H, Lee K. Clinical syndromes and management of intracerebral hemorrhage. Current Atherosclerosis Reports. 2012;**14**(4):307-313

[7] Auer RN, Sutherland GR. Primary intracerebral hemorrhage: Pathophysiology. Canadian Journal of Neurological Sciences. 2005;**32**(Suppl 2):S3-S12

[8] Kazui S, Naritomi H, Yamamoto H, Sawada T, Yamaguchi T. Enlargement of spontaneous intracerebral hemorrhage: Incidence and time course. Stroke. 1996;**27**(10):1783-1787

[9] Rønning P, Sorteberg W, Nakstad P, Russell D, Helseth E. Aspects of intracerebral hematomas: An update. Acta Neurologica Scandinavica. 2008;**118**(6):347-361

[10] Sonni S, Lioutas V, Selim M. New avenues for treatment of intracranial hemorrhage. Current Treatment Options in Cardiovascular Medicine. 2013;**16**(1):1-15

[11] Mayer S, Brun N, Begtrup K, Broderick J, Davis S, Diringer M, et al. Efficacy and safety of recombinant activated factor VII for acute intracerebral hemorrhage. New England Journal of Medicine. 2008;**358**(20):2127-2137

[12] Gulati D, Dua D, Torbey M. Hemostasis in intracranial hemorrhage. Frontiers in Neurology. 2017;**8**:80.

[13] Morgenstern L, Hemphill J, Anderson C, Becker K, Broderick J, Connolly E, et al. Guidelines for the management of spontaneous intracerebral hemorrhage: A guideline for healthcare professionals from the American Heart Association/American Stroke Association. Stroke. 2010;**41**(9):2108-2129

[14] Uyttenboogaart M, Jacobs B. Surgery for cerebral haemorrhage—STICH II trial. The Lancet. 2013;**382**(9902):1401

[15] WICH 2017. Brain Injury Outcomes [Internet]. 2017. Available from: http://braininjury-outcomes.com [Accessed: June 7, 2017]

Chapter 2

Intracerebral Hematoma

Shankar Ayyappan Kutty

Additional information is available at the end of the chapter

http://dx.doi.org/10.5772/66867

Abstract

Intracerebral hematoma occurs in about 35/100,000 population and the incidence is likely increase over the next few decades as the population ages. The most common causes are hypertension and amyloid angiopathy. Bleeds due to these two causes are classified as primary while all other causes, such as AVM bleeds, coagulopathies, and so on, are classified as secondary. Primary tissue damage due to the intracerebral hematoma is followed by edema, neuronal damage, and secondary damage due to cellular breakdown. Basal ganglia are the most common site of intracerebral hemorrhage, accounting for nearly 50% of cases. CT scan, CT angiogram, DSA, and MRI are the investigations of choice. The initial management is medical, with control of blood pressure and antiedema measures forming the mainstay of treatment. Surgical option includes external ventricular drainage, endoscopic evacuation of hematoma, craniotomy and evacuation of hematoma, and decompressive craniectomy and is usually reserved for patients who deteriorate while on treatment.

Keywords: intracerebral hematoma, management, guidelines

1. Epidemiology

Intracerebral hemorrhage (ICH) or hemorrhage within the brain parenchyma is the second most common cause of all cases of sudden neurological deficits following strokes and has the highest mortality amongst all varieties of stroke [1]. A study in 1993 [2] showed that 1-year survival following an ICH was 38% and this had improved to only 52% by 2009 [3]. In-hospital mortality has remained stable at around 34% over the last three decades [4], all of which makes prevention a cornerstone of treatment of this devastating disease. The incidence of ICH in the United States is estimated to be about 24.6/100,000 of person years, ranging from 1.8 to 129 per 100,000 person years [5] and this is likely to go up over the next few decades as the percentage of the elderly in the population increases.

One of the major risk factors identified with ICH has been that of race, with Asian populations being affected almost twice as much as other races. Whites appear to have a lower incidence when compared to nonwhites. The second risk factor to be identified was age, with those over 85 years of age having a 10-fold increase in the incidence of ICH compared to younger patients. Women were found to have a 15% lower chance of hemorrhages, but this was not statistically significant [6]. The single most important modifiable risk factor associated with ICH has undeniably been hypertension. A meta-analysis of 11 case control studies found the risk of bleeding in hypertensives to be 3.5 times above that in normotensives [7] while a multicentric case control study put the risk at nine times above that in normotensives in patients who had a blood pressure of over 160/90 mm Hg [8]. Even increases within the normal range of blood pressure have been associated with a linear increase in the risk of ICH [9].

Increased alcohol intake in the 24 hours preceding the onset of bleed as well as during the week prior to the ictus have been identified as independent risk factors for ICH [10] and the location of the hematoma in these patients tended to be lobar [11]. While high cholesterol levels have been associated with increased risk for ischaemic stroke, low cholesterol has been associated with an increased risk of cerebral micro bleeds and ICH. However, the exact association of different lipid fractions with this risk has yet to be elucidated [12]. Recent studies have shown that apolipoprotein E (APOE) ε2 and ε4 are independent risk factors for lobar ICH, which stands to reason considering their association with amyloidosis [13]. Tobacco smoking has been consistently associated with occlusive diseases such as coronary and peripheral vascular disease, as well as ischaemic stroke and subarachnoid hemorrhage, but its association with ICH is tenuous at best [14].

2. Etiology

ICH has been divided into primary and secondary varieties based on the underlying pathology. When no underlying pathology such as vascular malformation or coagulopathy is detected, and the primary cause of the bleed is due to rupture of small vessels in the brain, usually secondary to chronic damage from long-standing hypertension or cerebral amyloid angiopathy, the bleed is considered primary (**Figures 1** and **2**). Nearly 80% of all intracerebral hematoma cases fall into this category [15].

Chronically elevated blood pressure causes smooth cell hyperplasia in the cerebral arteries, followed by death of smooth muscle cells. There is also an increase in the stiffness of arterial walls in these patients, and this loss of elasticity may predispose to arterial rupture with sudden elevations in blood pressure. Electron microscopic studies have shown that most ruptures occur near the bifurcation of arteries, where there is degeneration of tunica media. This may be why most of the bleeds that occur in hypertension are located in deeper parts of the brain [16, 17]. Cerebral amyloid angiopathy, in contrast, features amyloid deposition in the leptomeningeal and intraparenchymal cortical vessels, resulting in superficial or lobar hemorrhages. Patients with amyloidosis are more likely to be older (over 60 years of age) and have hematoma sizes greater than 30 cc while those with hypertension are younger and have hematoma volumes less

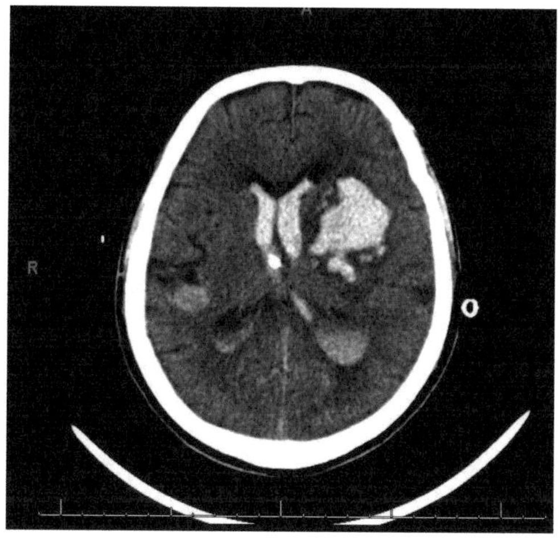

Figure 1. Hypertensive left ganglionic hematoma with IVH.

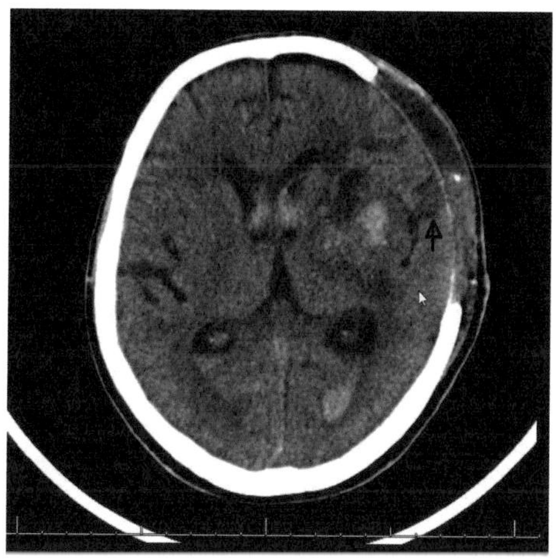

Figure 2. Same patient as in **Figure 1**, after surgical evacuation of hematoma following neurological deterioration. The black arrow shows widening of Sylvian fissure, which was split to approach the hematoma from its most superficial area. The bone flap was not replaced due to severe brain swelling.

than 30 cc [18]. A history of recurrent episodes of intracranial bleeds is likely to favor a diagnosis of cerebral amyloid angiopathy. It should, however, be borne in mind that these characteristics are nonspecific and need to be confirmed by histopathology if possible [19].

Bleeding from vascular malformations such as arteriovenous malformation (**Figure 3**), cavernous angiomas, and dural arteriovenous (AV) fistulae, hemorrhagic conversion of an ischemic stroke, bleeding from intraparenchymal tumors, ICH occurring in patients with bleeding diathesis and in those taking anticoagulants (**Figure 4**) all come into the category of secondary ICH [20]. Tumor bleeds typically occur in metastases, such as melanoma, choriocarcinoma, renal carcinoma, or thyroid carcinoma, and from high grade gliomas [21]. Aneurysmal bleeds

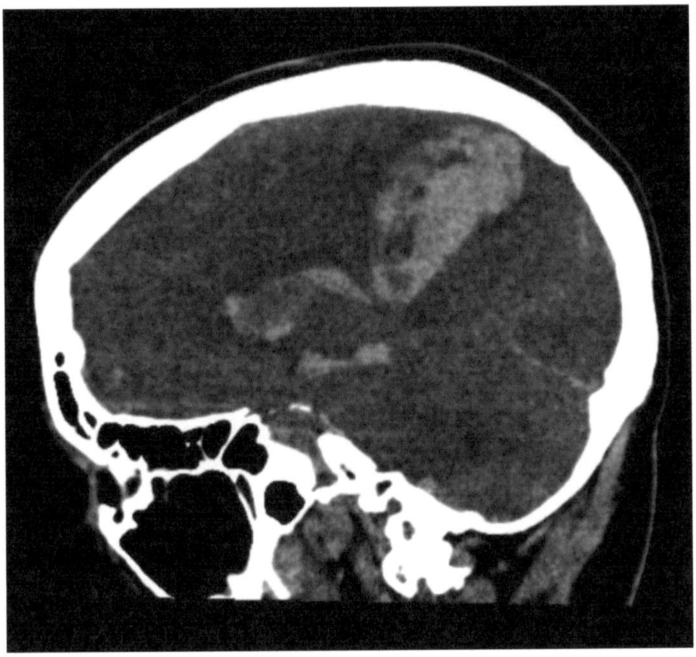

Figure 3. Large lobar hematoma with IVH due to a vascular malformation.

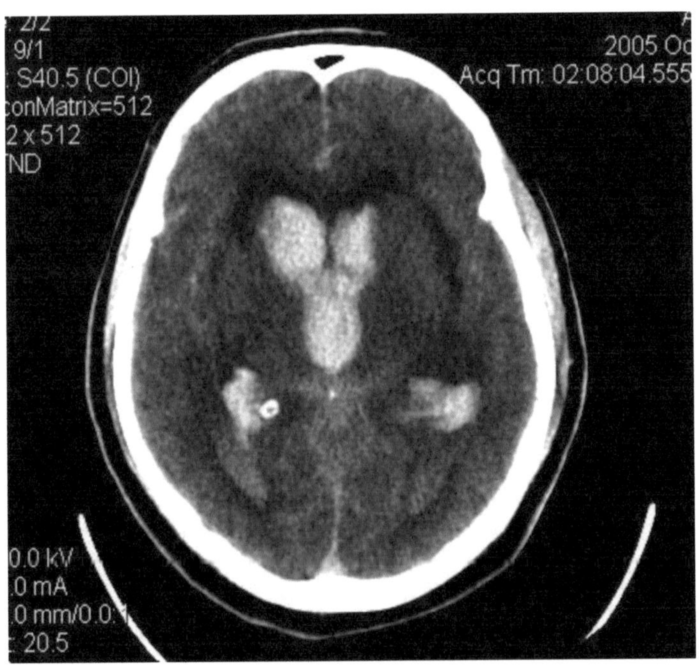

Figure 4. Isolated IVH in an anticoagulated patient.

http://dx.doi.org/10.5772/66867

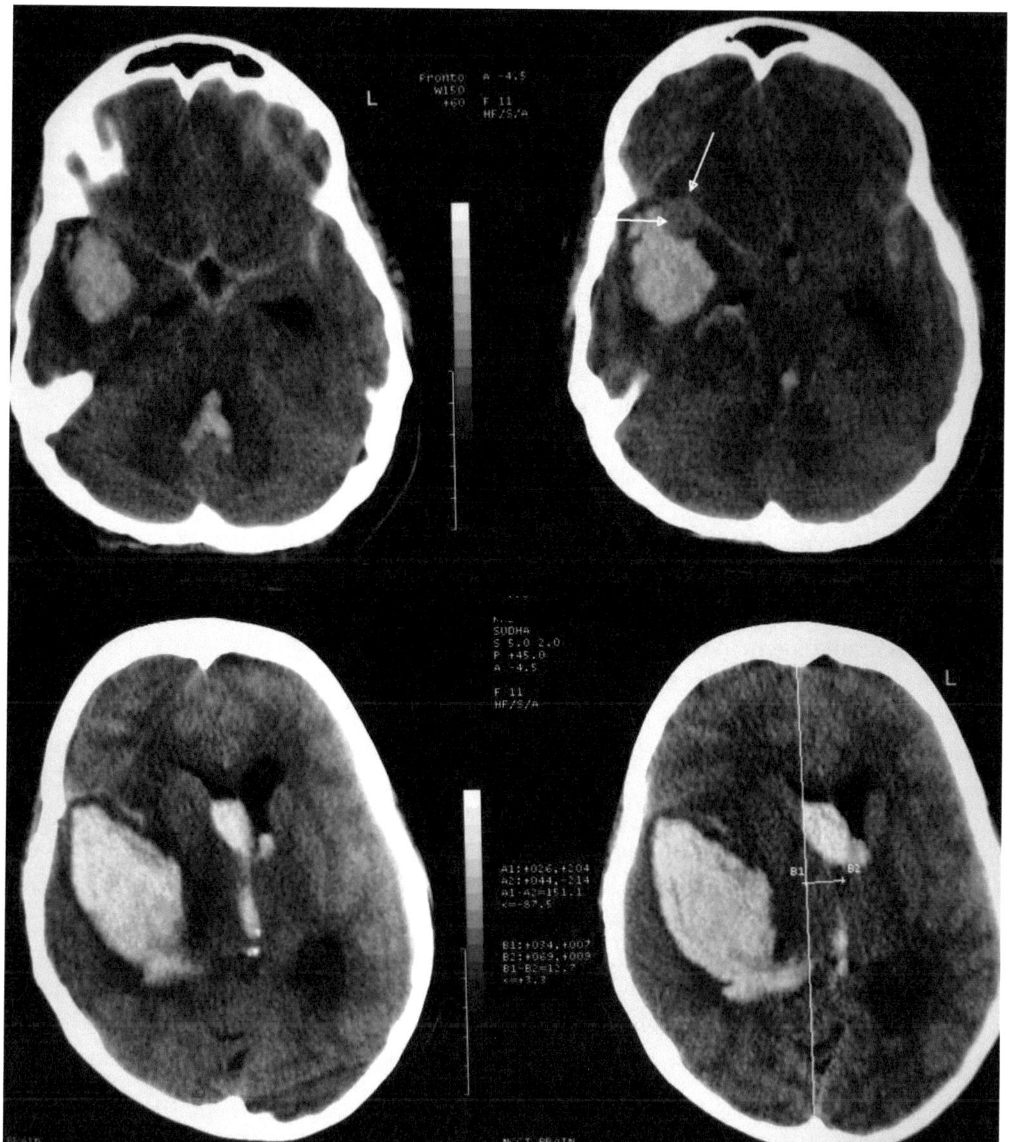

Figure 5. This patient had a bleed which looked like a ganglionic hematoma with IVH, but closer observation showed a partially thrombosed MCA aneurysm (white arrows, top right).

(**Figure 5**) may sometimes present with an intraparenchymal component and an ICH may occasionally be the result of a sinus thrombosis [22]. Recently, patients with hepatitis C infection have been identified as having a higher risk of ICH compared to a control group without HCV infection. The risk was higher in younger patients and increased with increasing severity of the viral infection [23]. Drug abuse, especially cocaine use, has been found to cause an increased incidence of subcortical hemorrhages with intraventricular extension and these patients have a poorer prognosis when compared to nondrug users with spontaneous ICH [24]. Patients or oral warfarin have an 8- to 14-fold increase in the risk of ICH compared to the normal population, but the risk appears to be lower in those being treated with newer anticoagulants such as dabigatran [25, 26].

3. Pathophysiology

Intracerebral hemorrhage results in primary damage due to the injury to neural tissues. This is followed by secondary damage resulting from increased intracranial pressure as well as the presence of intraparenchymal blood. The secondary damage occurs through several pathways that run concurrently, eventually leading to the loss of the blood brain barrier and severe cerebral edema resulting in extensive cellular lysis. As in traumatic brain injury, early removal of the hematoma and cellular debris, either by surgical removal of the clot or by the action of the inflammatory cells such as microglia and macrophages, help to reduce the extent of secondary damage [27, 28]. Animal studies have shown that perihematoma edema can be divided into three phases: immediate (up to 24 h after hemorrhage), intermediate (from 24 h to 5 days), and late (beyond 5 days) [29]. The immediate edema results from osmotically active proteins accumulating in the extravascular compartment and can be seen on histological studies, but not on imaging. Intracerebral hemorrhage results in primary damage due to the injury to neural tissues. This is followed by secondary damage resulting from increased intracranial pressure as well as the presence of intraparenchymal blood. The secondary damage occurs through several pathways that run concurrently, eventually leading to the loss of the blood brain barrier and severe cerebral edema resulting in extensive cellular lysis. As in traumatic brain injury, early removal of the hematoma and cellular debris, either by surgical removal of the clot or by the action of the inflammatory cells such as microglia and macrophages, help to reduce the extent of secondary damage [30]. Red cell destruction due to activation of the clotting cascade releases thrombin which again causes disruption of the blood brain barrier, failure of the sodium pump, and increase in the edema [31, 32]. This intermediate edema can be visualized radiologically. The late cerebral edema results from oxidative damage due free radical release which is a result of cellular destruction and hemoglobin breakdown.

Several additional pathways for cellular damage following intracerebral hemorrhage have been advocated, such as apoptosis or programmed cell death associated with the expression of nuclear factor-kB in neuronal nuclei [33] and breakdown of extravasated heme into bilirubin and bilirubin oxidation products, which activate microglia. The microglia then activate leucocyte adhesion molecules on endothelial walls, leading to an influx of leucocytes into the brain. The activated microglia produce cytokines which along with the leucocytes mediate further cell injury [34].

The commonest site for an intracerebral hematoma is the basal ganglia, with the putamen being the preferred location. Nearly 50% of all ICH cases involve in the basal ganglia, followed by the thalamus, pons, cerebral white matter, and brainstem. The source of bleeding is usually a Charcot-Bouchard micro-aneurysm, arising from either the lenticulostriate arteries in case of putaminal bleeds or thalamoperforators in case of the thalamic bleeds. The paramedian branches of the basilar artery are the source for basilar and cerebellar hemorrhages [35].

http://dx.doi.org/10.5772/66867

4. Presentation

The clinical presentation of intracerebral hemorrhage depends on the location of the bleed and its size. Smaller bleeds in non-eloquent areas may present with headache, nausea, and vomiting. Larger hemorrhages into the frontal lobe may be associated with contralateral hemiparesis, mainly involving the upper limbs, and aphasia if the dominant lobe is involved. Parietal lobe involvement causes contralateral hemisensory impairment with mild hemiparesis and cognitive impairment. Occipital hematomas may present with pain in the ipsilateral eye and contralateral homonymous hemianopia. Dominant temporal lobe involvement causes Wernicke's aphasia which may be associated with poor auditory comprehension, while nondominant temporal lobe hemorrhage may be asymptomatic unless it is large enough to cause symptoms due to the mass effect. Putaminal hemorrhages may present with a range of symptomatology, from minimal pure motor deficits on the contralateral side to severe sensorimotor impairment, aphasia, neglect, gaze deviation, and impaired level of consciousness. These patients have a gradual deterioration in clinical symptoms from the time of onset with a 30-day mortality as high as 50%, but only a small percentage has headache as a presenting symptom [36]. In contrast, nearly 30% of patients with a thalamic bleed present with headache. They have hemisensory disturbances that are out of proportion to the minimal weakness. Significant weakness may be found when the hematoma extends into the internal capsule and associated eye signs indicate involvement of the midbrain.

Tanaka et al. [37] found that when compared to putaminal hemorrhages, thalamic hemorrhages were associated with a more pronounced reduction in cerebral blood flow (CBF)

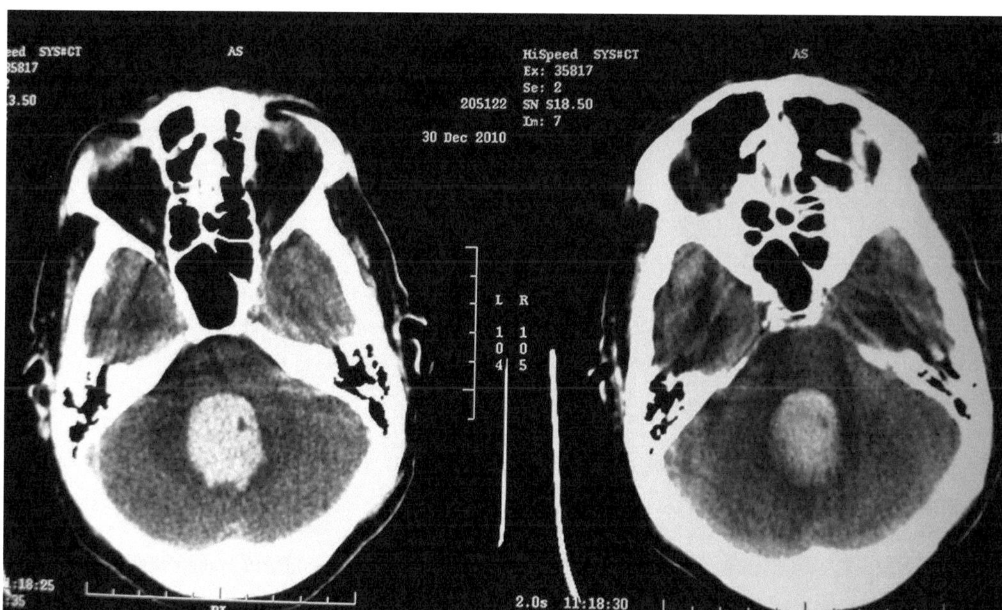

Figure 6. Preoperative images of a vermian hematoma with intraventricular extension in a patient with hemophilia.

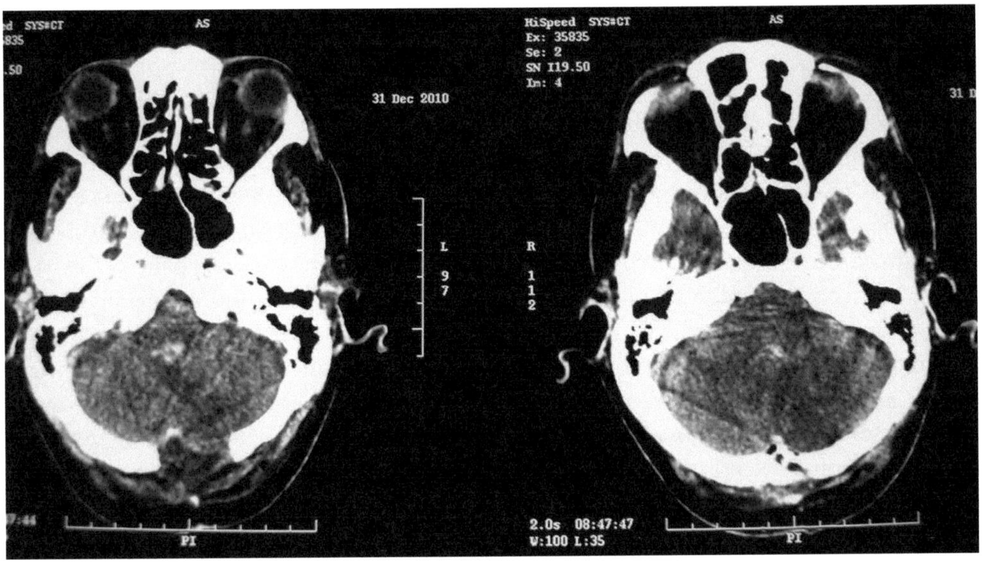

Figure 7. Postoperative images of a vermian hematoma with intraventricular extension in a patient with hemophilia.

bilaterally, even though their hematoma volumes were much smaller. They hypothesized that the reduction of CBF may be secondary to metabolic depression due to transneuronal or functional depression ("diaschisis"). The metabolic depression in thalamic hemorrhages is more extensive and persistent than in putaminal hemorrhages, which probably accounts for the reduced CBF and worse outcome in thalamic hemorrhages. While several studies have quoted a size of 3.3 cm as a determinant for survival in patients with thalamic hemorrhages [38–40] in a prospective trial that included 100 patients there were three survivors with hematomas larger than 3.3 cm who were able to lead independent lives [41]. However, sizes of the hematoma and intraventricular extension were two major factors that were found to correlate with the eventual outcome.

Cerebellar ICH may present with limb ataxia, ipsilateral gaze palsy, cranial nerve deficits such as an abducens or peripheral facial palsy, and nonspecific symptoms like headache and vomiting. In a series of 56 patients, Ott et al. found that nearly three-fourth of the patients had one of the first three signs described [42]. As in other types of ICH, intraventricular extension, initial GCS, and older age were associated with a poor prognosis in patients with cerebellar ICH (**Figures 6** and **7**) [43].

5. Evaluation

A plain computerized tomography (CT) scan of the brain is the standard investigation performed in all suspected intracranial pathologies which present as an emergency. In cases of ICH, CT scan will usually reveal a hyperdense lesion within the brain parenchyma, with possible intraventricular or subarachnoid components. The latter typically occurs with anterior communicating or middle cerebral artery aneurysms.

The volume of the hematoma can be calculated by the modified ellipsoid volume calculation where the anteroposterior (A), right to left (B), and cranio-caudal lengths of the clot (C) are measured. The last (that is, C) is calculated by counting the number of slices in which the clot is seen and multiplying it by the slice thickness. The formula (A×B×C)/2 can then be used to calculate the clot volume [44]. On multivariate analysis in several studies, initial Glasgow Coma Scale score, hematoma volume, and an infratentorial location of hemorrhage were found to correlate strongly with the outcome of intracerebral hematoma. Univariate analysis had also implicated higher initial and 48-h maximum glucose concentrations, and higher percentage of ICH expansion as being significantly associated with poor functional outcome at hospital discharge. In anticoagulated patients, the initial INR or the time to INR correction did not affect the outcome [45].

Magnetic resonance imaging (MRI) is rarely the investigation of choice in the acute scenario due to various reasons. A complete study requires much more time than a CT scan and the spontaneous movements of a partially obtunded patient may cause imaging artefacts and significantly prolong the imaging time. If the patient worsens clinically while undergoing imaging, it may be difficult to access him immediately. Initially, it was felt that small amounts of hyperacute blood were difficult to visualize in many imaging sequences, but a study by Linfante et al. showed that MRI scans were capable of demonstrating a hyperacute bleed within 2 h of symptom onset [46]. An advantage of MRI is the ability of gradient echo sequences to distinguish hemorrhages of varying ages, which is extremely useful in amyloid angiopathy and cavernous angiomas.

While initial investigators believed that the progressive neurological deterioration that occurred in the hours following an intracerebral hemorrhage were due to the mass effect of the hematoma, radiological studies have shown that early hematoma growth occurs in up to 38% of all patients with ICH [47]. This has led to efforts to identify the factors that promote rehemorrhage, so as to identify the patients at risk of deterioration, as well as to develop management strategies to prevent a rebleed. The major risk factors for a rebleed include uncontrolled hypertension with a systolic blood pressure more than 195 mm Hg, a previous infarction at the site of the hemorrhage, alcoholism which predisposes to liver disease and which in turn leads to coagulopathies, anticoagulant use, high white cell count, and hyperthermia [48]. Contrast extravasation on CT angiography was found to correlate well with the risk of rehemorrhage [49]. The presence of tiny enhancing foci, known as the "spot sign" on axial images of a 3D CT angiogram has been reported to be associated with a higher risk of hematoma expansion [50]. This correlation was found to be true especially when the Hounsfield units (HU) of these foci were in the range of 192.12 ± 45.97 while patients with spot signs having a lower HU of 151.10 ± 25 did not suffer from a hematoma expansion [51]. The surgical trial in intracerebral hemorrhage (STICH trial) introduced the concept of a prognostication score for ICH, which was calculated using the equation (10 × admission GCS) – age (years) – (0.64 × clot volume (ml)) [52].

If there is a suspicion of a vascular anomaly as the main cause of the hemorrhage, and if the CT angiogram is noncontributory, a catheter angiogram (cerebral DSA) should be considered.

6. Medical management

The optimum treatment for intracerebral hemorrhage is an area of ongoing research and changing guidelines (**Table 1**). While the STICH trial went some way in answering some of the questions regarding the role of surgery, it also raised a number of issues which are yet to be resolved [53]. The initial, prehospital and emergency room management for patients with ICH is the same as those for patients with ischemic stroke and was elucidated in the guidelines published by the American Heart Association (AHA) and the American Stroke Association in 2013. A severity score should be calculated as soon as possible, so as to enable prognostication (**Tables 2** and **3**). If facilities for stroke care are not available in the hospital, the patient should be transferred to a tertiary care center as early as possible.

No.	Problem	Recommendation	Class of evidence
1	Initial presentation in emergency	Perform baseline ICH severity score	I
2	Differentiate between ischemic and hemorrhagic stroke	CT or MRI scan	I
3	Possibility of hematoma expansion	Contrast CT and CT angiogram to be considered	IIb
4	Vascular anomaly	CT or MR angiograms (arterial/venous studies) and DSA to be considered	IIa
5	Management of coagulation defects	Correct coagulopathy or thrombocytopenia with appropriate therapy	I
6	Patients on vitamin K antagonists (VKA)	Stop VKA, give intravenous vitamin K	I
7		Fresh frozen plasma (FFP) or prothrombin complex concentrates (PCC)	IIb
8	Patients on heparin	Protamine sulphate	IIb
9	Patients on newer anticoagulants	PCC, factor VIII inhibitor bypassing activity (FEIBA) or rFVIIa, hemodialysis and activated charcoal if drug was ingested within 2 h	IIb
10	Prevention of deep venous thrombosis (DVT)	Intermittent pneumatic compression	I
		Low molecular weight heparin to be considered after 1–4 days once cessation of hematoma expansion is documented	IIb
11	Established DVT	IVC filter or systemic anticoagulation	IIa
12	Hypertension (systolic BP 150–220 mm Hg) without contraindication for acute lowering of BP	Lower SBP to 140 mm Hg	Ia
	Hypertension (SBP > 220 mm Hg)	Aggressive reduction of SBP	IIb

No.	Problem	Recommendation	Class of evidence
13	High blood sugar	Control adequately, avoiding hypoglycemia	I
14	Fever	Control adequately	IIb
15	Seizures	Clinical seizures and abnormal EEG in patients with altered mental status should be treated	I
		Continuous EEG monitoring in patients with altered mental status that is out of proportion to extent of brain injury	IIa
16	Concurrent cardiac events	ECG and cardiac enzymes to be checked	IIa
17	Hydrocephalus	Ventricular drainage	IIa
18	GCS less than or equal to 8, presence of IVH	ICP monitoring, maintain CPP at 50–70 mm Hg	IIb
19	IVH	Intraventricular rtPA-efficacy uncertain	IIb
20	Cerebellar hematoma, neurological deterioration	Surgical evacuation	I
21	Supratentorial ICH, neurological deterioration	Surgical evacuation	IIb
		Decompressive craniectomy	IIb
		Minimally invasive clot evacuation-efficacy uncertain	IIb
22	Aspiration pneumonia	Screen for dysphagia before starting oral feeds	I

Table 1. Evidence-based recommendations on management.

Component	Value	Points
Glasgow Coma Scale (total score)	3–4	2
	5–12	1
	13–15	0
Intracerebral hematoma volume	≥30 cm^3	1
	<30 cm^3	0
Intraventricular hemorrhage	Present	1
	Absent	0
Origin of intracerebral hematoma	Infratentorial	1
	Supratentorial	0
Age	≥80 years	1
	<80 years	0

Table 2. ICH severity score [89].

Total ICH score (points)	Mortality rate (%)
0	0
1	13
2	26
3	72
4	97
5–6	100

Table 3. The total ICH score obtained by adding all the component scores from **Table 1** can be used to prognosticate the mortality as given below.

The patient has to be admitted into a dedicated stroke unit or an intensive care unit, and invasive (arterial) blood pressure monitoring should be instituted as soon as possible for control of hypertension. The INTERACT2 trial showed a significantly better outcome for patients whose systolic blood pressure (SBP) was less than 140 mm Hg compared against a group where the SBP was less than 180 mm Hg [54]. Therefore, an SBP of 140 mm Hg should be targeted for all patients admitted with ICH. If multiple, long-term, intravenous access is anticipated, a multi-lumen central venous line can be inserted if the coagulation profile is normal.

Patients with a low Glasgow Coma Scale score who are not candidates for early surgery may need intracranial pressure monitoring. Using an intraventricular catheter for the same has the dual advantage of monitoring pressure and allowing drainage of CSF, for countering acute rise in intracranial pressure and in cases of obstructive hydrocephalus due to intraventricular hemorrhage. The intraventricular blood may frequently block the catheter, which can be overcome by using a thrombolytic agent such as 1 mg of tissue plasminogen activator (tPA) given through the catheter, following which the catheter is clamped for 30 min. This can be repeated every 8 hours until the third and the fourth ventricles are cleared of blood on CT or until a maximum cumulative dose of 20 mg rtPA is reached [55]. Ventricular catheters, however, are associated with a higher risk of parenchymal bleeds and infections, and this has to be borne in mind while choosing the type of ICP monitoring. In patients with coagulation disorders, the coagulation should be corrected and if the patient is on antiplatelet drugs, platelet transfusion administered prior to catheter insertion [56].

As the medical management of ICH aims primarily to reduce the intracranial pressure, the tenets of management have been borrowed from the experience gained in treating traumatic brain injury. Mannitol has been the mainstay in the management of raised ICP for a long time, but problems such as rebound phenomenon have led to the increasing use of hypertonic saline (23.4%) for the same purpose [57]. Both the drugs can be used in patients with ICH but the latter may be more effective [58].

Though initial trials with recombinant activated factor VII (rFVIIa) showed promise in limiting the hematoma size following early administration of the drug to patients with intracerebral hemorrhage, this was not borne out in phase three trials [59, 60] Furthermore, the use of rFVIIa has been associated with an increased incidence of thromboembolic events compared to placebo (7% vs. 2%) and as such the medication is not recommended in noncoagulopathic patients (**Table 4**) [56].

Therapy	Class of evidence
rFVIIa for VKA reversal	III
Prophylactic anticonvulsants	III
Intraventricular drainage in patients with cerebellar hematoma, brainstem compression	III
Early surgery for clot evacuation in a stable patient	IIb

Table 4. Therapies not indicated in ICH.

A vast majority of patients with ICH have fever during the postictal period and the incidence is higher in those with intraventricular hemorrhage. The duration of fever correlates inversely with the patient outcome. Furthermore, cooling the body has been reported to reduce the perihematoma edema, and hence body temperature needs to be controlled with medicines or external cooling after an ICH [61–63].

Almost all patients admitted in the ICU after an intracranial bleed have stress induced hyperglycemia. This may result in loss of control of blood sugars in a diabetic, or high blood sugars in a nondiabetic, both of which are associated with a poor outcome in patients with supratentorial ICH [64]. A study suggested improved clinical outcomes with tight control of blood sugar to the range of 80–110 mg%, but this was found to cause occasional hypoglycemia resulting in increased mortality [65, 66]. As such, no specific target is recommended for blood sugar control in these patients and the broad recommendation that both hypo- and hyperglycemia need to be avoided can probably be met by trying to maintain the blood sugar levels in the range of 120–150 mg%, at least till new evidence is available.

Up to 16% of patients have seizures after an ICH and the incidence is higher in those with lobar bleeds, probably due to the cortical involvement in this cohort of patients. While the incidence of seizures in these patients can be reduced by use of prophylactic anticonvulsants, their use has not been associated with any change in long-term clinical outcome or mortality [67–69]. Though some studies had linked the use of antiseizure drugs, particularly phenytoin, to increased death and disability, probably due to their sedative and cardiovascular side effects, a recent study found no such correlation [70–72]. A study of sodium valproate showed no difference in the rate of new onset seizures in patients given either a placebo (22.2%) or the drug (19.5%) [73]. Therefore, use of prophylactic anticonvulsants is not recommended at present.

The co-occurrence of myocardial infarction and ischemic stroke has been well documented, and Sandhu et al. found that 15% of patients admitted to the ICU who had an elevated troponin I level in the first 24 h, and that is contributed to an increased mortality [74]. A large meta-analysis of stroke patients put the annual risk of MI at 2.2% for these patients [75]. A preventive protocol including cardiac enzymes, ECG, and echocardiogram should be in place for the management of patients with ICH.

Many patients with intracerebral hemorrhage have an associated coagulopathy or platelet dysfunction, either due to an underlying disease such as factor deficiency or due to the use of anticoagulant/antiplatelet medications. The presence of such a coagulopathy must be identified and corrective measures taken as soon as the patient is admitted, in order to prevent hematoma expansion. The detailed management of patients on oral anticoagulants can be obtained from the guidelines published by the American College of Chest Physicians [76].

Intraventricular hemorrhage associated with ICH has been consistently associated with a worsening of the eventual patient outcome. While an external ventricular drain is useful in draining the blood and treating the obstructive hydrocephalus produced due to obstruction of the ventricular pathway by blood clots, this treatment is not very effective in practice due to the propensity of blood clots to also block the catheter. The use of local fibrinolytic agents was promoted to overcome this problem. The CLEAR-IVH (clot lysis: evaluating accelerated resolution of IVH) trial [77] showed that there was a significant reduction in the incidence of catheter blockage and duration of catheter insertion in patients given intraventricular rtPA. They had a lower incidence of permanent CSF diversion procedures, but also suffered a higher incidence of rehemorrhage [78, 79]. An alternative to the use of intraventricular catheters is the endoscopic clearance of the intraventricular hemorrhage. While studies have not shown any improvement in mortality or neurological outcome, patients who underwent endoscopic clot evacuation have been reported to have a lower requirement of permanent CSF diversion procedures [80].

7. Surgical management

The exact role that surgery plays in the management of ICH remains shrouded in controversy, mainly due to the multitude of factors and the heterogeneity of patients that present with ICH. The largest studies that looked at the benefit of early surgery for patients with supratentorial ICH did not show any benefit compared to medical management, but detailed analysis showed that two subgroups of patients had a better prognosis with surgery. The first were those with lobar hemorrhages within 1 cm of the cortical surface and the second were those who were assigned a poor prognosis at the time of presentation, using a formula devised for the study.

The ideal surgical procedure is also open to question, with the reported procedures including craniotomy and evacuation of the hematoma, decompressive craniectomy, minimally invasive clot evacuation with the use of rtPA (MISTIE II), stereotactic aspiration of the clot and needle aspiration of the basal ganglionic hematoma [81–84].

There is more clarity in cases of infratentorial hematoma, with most surgeons in agreement that pontine hemorrhages are best managed conservatively (**Figure 8**). This is due to the difficulty in surgically accessing the brainstem, the morbidity associated with surgery on the brain stem and the high mortality associated with these hemorrhages. However, it has been noted

http://dx.doi.org/10.5772/66867

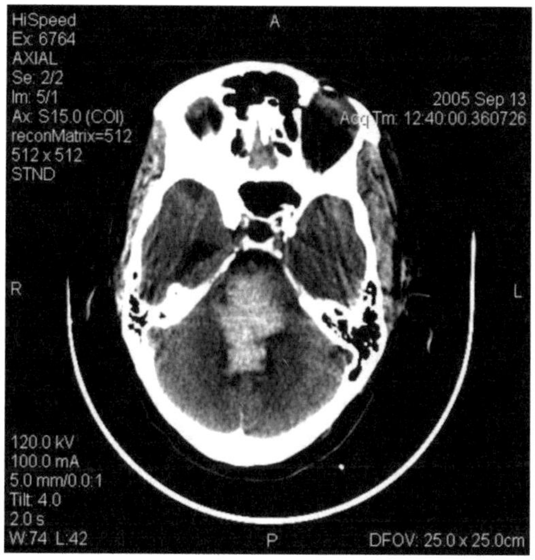

Figure 8. Large hypertensive pontine hemorrhage destroying the entire brainstem.

that patients with bleeding cavernous malformations have a much better outcome than those in whom the cause of hemorrhage is uncontrolled hypertension, and this subgroup may merit surgery [85]. On the other hand, most patients with cerebellar hemorrhages warrant early surgery, especially when the clot volume is more than 3 cm. This is due to the direct compression of brainstem caused by even small infratentorial hemorrhages, due to the small volume of the posterior fossa and the propensity of these bleeds to cause obstructive hydrocephalus. Insertion of external ventricular drain to treat the hydrocephalus may seem like a logical move, but patients thus treated have had a worse prognosis due to the incidence of reverse transtentorial herniation following decompression of the ventricles [86, 87].

While performing a craniotomy for evacuation of ICH, a few points have to be kept in mind [88].

1. Position the patient so that a vertical track from the surface will lead to the hematoma. This will reduce the chances of the surgeon becoming disoriented and missing the hematoma.

2. In putaminal hemorrhages, the shortest track will often involve dissecting the Sylvian and performing the corticectomy in the insula (see **Figure 2**).

3. In deep-seated hematomas, use intraoperative ultrasound or neuronavigation to find the shortest track to the clot to avoid excessive damage to normal brain.

4. When there is a large hematoma abutting the Sylvian fissure, a preoperative angiography (CTA or DSA) should be done to exclude a middle cerebral artery aneurysm (see **Figure 5**).

5. After obtaining hemostasis, increase the blood pressure by 20–30 mm Hg above the baseline and ensure there is no bleeding, so as to reduce the risk of rebleed.

6. In most cases, the bone flap can be safely replaced as the brain will be lax once the hematoma is evacuated.

8. Conclusion

The goal of treatment in patients with ICH is very similar to that in traumatic brain injury, namely, to prevent further damage. This can be achieved by preventing the expansion of the hematoma, reducing ischemic and hypoxic damage, removal of the hematoma, and management of hydrocephalus when appropriate and effective rehabilitation. Primary prevention by controlling hypertension should be a goal of national healthcare programs. Many of the strategies used in the management of these patients is in a state of constant flux since studies on the subject wind up raising more questions than they answer. It is up to the physicians to constantly update themselves on the best management protocols for these patients, and to devote some time to clinical research that will shed more light on this devastating disease.

Author details

Shankar Ayyappan Kutty

Address all correspondence to: shankar.ayyappan@nmc.ae

NMC Specialty Hospital, Abu Dhabi, United Arab Emirates

References

[1] Feigin VL, Lawes CMM, Bennett DA, Barker-Collo SL, Parag V. Worldwide stroke incidence and early case fatality reported in 56 population-based studies: a systematic review. Lancet Neurol. 2009 Apr;8(4):355-69.

[2] Dennis MS, Burn JP, Sandercock PA, Bamford JM, Wade DT, Warlow CP. Long-term survival after first-ever stroke: the oxfordshire community stroke project. Stroke J Cereb Circ. 1993 Jun;24(6):796-800.

[3] Zia E, Engström G, Svensson PJ, Norrving B, Pessah-Rasmussen H. Three-year survival and stroke recurrence rates in patients with primary intracerebral hemorrhage. Stroke J Cereb Circ. 2009 Nov;40(11):3567-73.

[4] Rincon F, Mayer SA. The epidemiology of intracerebral hemorrhage in the United States from 1979 to 2008. Neurocrit Care. 2013 Aug;19(1):95-102.

[5] Ikram MA, Wieberdink RG, Koudstaal PJ. International epidemiology of intracerebral hemorrhage. Curr Atheroscler Rep. 2012 Aug;14(4):300-6.

[6] van Asch CJ, Luitse MJ, Rinkel GJ, van der Tweel I, Algra A, Klijn CJ. Incidence, case fatality, and functional outcome of intracerebral haemorrhage over time, according to age, sex, and ethnic origin: a systematic review and meta-analysis. Lancet Neurol. 2010 Feb;9(2):167-76.

[7] Ariesen MJ, Claus SP, Rinkel GJE, Algra A. Risk factors for intracerebral hemorrhage in the general population: a systematic review. Stroke J Cereb Circ. 2003 Aug;34(8):2060-5.

[8] O'Donnell MJ, Xavier D, Liu L, Zhang H, Chin SL, Rao-Melacini P, et al. Risk factors for ischaemic and intracerebral haemorrhagic stroke in 22 countries (the interstroke study): a case-control study. Lancet Lond Engl. 2010 Jul 10;376(9735):112-23.

[9] Leppälä JM, Virtamo J, Fogelholm R, Albanes D, Heinonen OP. Different risk factors for different stroke subtypes: association of blood pressure, cholesterol, and antioxidants. Stroke J Cereb Circ. 1999 Dec;30(12):2535-40.

[10] Juvela S, Hillbom M, Palomäki H. Risk factors for spontaneous intracerebral hemorrhage. Stroke J Cereb Circ. 1995 Sep;26(9):1558-64.

[11] Monforte R, Estruch R, Graus F, Nicolas JM, Urbano-Marquez A. High ethanol consumption as risk factor for intracerebral hemorrhage in young and middle-aged people. Stroke J Cereb Circ. 1990 Nov;21(11):1529-32.

[12] Wieberdink RG, Poels MMF, Vernooij MW, Koudstaal PJ, Hofman A, van der Lugt A, et al. Serum lipid levels and the risk of intracerebral hemorrhage: the Rotterdam study. Arterioscler Thromb Vasc Biol. 2011 Dec;31(12):2982-9.

[13] Biffi A, Sonni A, Anderson CD, Kissela B, Jagiella JM, Schmidt H, et al. Variants at APOE influence risk of deep and lobar intracerebral hemorrhage. Ann Neurol. 2010 Dec;68(6):934-43.

[14] Paul SL, Thrift AG, Donnan GA. Smoking as a crucial independent determinant of stroke. Tob Induc Dis. 2004 Jun 15;2(1):7.

[15] Sutherland GR, Auer RN. Primary intracerebral hemorrhage. J Clin Neurosci Off J Neurosurg Soc Australas. 2006 Jun;13(5):511-7.

[16] Campbell GJ, Roach MR. Fenestrations in the internal elastic lamina at bifurcations of human cerebral arteries. Stroke J Cereb Circ. 1981 Aug;12(4):489-96.

[17] Acampa M, Guideri F, Di Donato I, Tassi R, Marotta G, Lo Giudice G, et al. Arterial stiffness in patients with deep and lobar intracerebral hemorrhage. J Stroke. 2014 Sep;16(3):184-8.

[18] Ritter MA, Droste DW, Hegedüs K, Szepesi R, Nabavi DG, Csiba L, et al. Role of cerebral amyloid angiopathy in intracerebral hemorrhage in hypertensive patients. Neurology. 2005 Apr 12;64(7):1233-7.

[19] Lang EW, Ren Ya Z, Preul C, Hugo HH, Hempelmann RG, Buhl R, et al. Stroke pattern interpretation: the variability of hypertensive versus amyloid angiopathy hemorrhage. Cerebrovasc Dis Basel Switz. 2001 Aug;12(2):121-30.

[20] Sahni R, Weinberger J. Management of intracerebral hemorrhage. Vasc Health Risk Manag. 2007 Oct;3(5):701-9.

[21] Kondziolka D, Lunsford LD, Kestle JR. The natural history of cerebral cavernous malformations. J Neurosurg. 1995 Nov;83(5):820-4.

[22] Canhão P, Ferro JM, Lindgren AG, Bousser M-G, Stam J, Barinagarrementeria F, et al. Causes and predictors of death in cerebral venous thrombosis. Stroke J Cereb Circ. 2005 Aug;36(8):1720-5.

[23] Tseng CH, Muo CH, Hsu CY, Kao CH. Increased risk of intracerebral hemorrhage among patients with hepatitis C virus infection. Medicine (Baltimore). 2015 Nov;94(46):e2132.

[24] Martin-Schild S, Albright KC, Hallevi H, Barreto AD, Philip M, Misra V, et al. Intracerebral hemorrhage in cocaine users. Stroke J Cereb Circ. 2010 Apr;41(4):680-4.

[25] Franke CL, de Jonge J, van Swieten JC, Op de Coul AA, van Gijn J. Intracerebral hematomas during anticoagulant treatment. Stroke J Cereb Circ. 1990 May;21(5):726-30.

[26] Schulman S, Kearon C, Kakkar AK, Mismetti P, Schellong S, Eriksson H, et al. Dabigatran versus warfarin in the treatment of acute venous thromboembolism. N Engl J Med. 2009 Dec 10;361(24):2342-52.

[27] Qureshi AI, Mendelow AD, Hanley DF. Intracerebral haemorrhage. Lancet Lond Engl. 2009 May 9;373(9675):1632-44.

[28] Aronowski J, Zhao X. Molecular pathophysiology of cerebral hemorrhage: secondary brain injury. Stroke J Cereb Circ. 2011 Jun;42(6):1781-6.

[29] Wagner KR, Xi G, Hua Y, Kleinholz M, de Courten-Myers GM, Myers RE. Early metabolic alterations in edematous perihematomal brain regions following experimental intracerebral hemorrhage. J Neurosurg. 1998 Jun;88(6):1058-65.

[30] Wu G, Sun S, Sheng F, Wang L, Wang F. Perihematomal glutamate level is associated with the blood–brain barrier disruption in a rabbit model of intracerebral hemorrhage. SpringerPlus [Internet]. 2013 Jul 30 [cited 2016 Sep 9];2. Available from: http://www.ncbi.nlm.nih.gov/pmc/articles/PMC3738910/

[31] Lee KR, Kawai N, Kim S, Sagher O, Hoff JT. Mechanisms of edema formation after intracerebral hemorrhage: effects of thrombin on cerebral blood flow, blood-brain barrier permeability, and cell survival in a rat model. J Neurosurg. 1997 Feb;86(2):272-8.

[32] Xi G, Hua Y, Bhasin RR, Ennis SR, Keep RF, Hoff JT. Mechanisms of edema formation after intracerebral hemorrhage: effects of extravasated red blood cells on blood flow and blood-brain barrier integrity. Stroke J Cereb Circ. 2001 Dec 1;32(12):2932-8.

[33] Hickenbottom SL, Grotta JC, Strong R, Denner LA, Aronowski J. Nuclear factor-kappaB and cell death after experimental intracerebral hemorrhage in rats. Stroke J Cereb Circ. 1999 Nov;30(11):2472-8.

[34] Loftspring MC, Hansen C, Clark JF. A novel brain injury mechanism after intracerebral hemorrhage: the interaction between heme products and the immune system. Med Hypotheses. 2010 Jan;74(1):63-6.

[35] Aguilar MI, Brott TG. Update in intracerebral hemorrhage. The Neurohospitalist. 2011 Jul;1(3):148-59.

[36] Little KM, Alexander MJ. Medical versus surgical therapy for spontaneous intracranial hemorrhage. Neurosurg Clin N Am. 2002 Jul;13(3):339-47.

[37] Tanaka A, Yoshinaga S, Nakayama Y, Kimura M, Tomonaga M. Cerebral blood flow and clinical outcome in patients with thalamic hemorrhages: a comparison with putaminal hemorrhages. J Neurol Sci. 1996 Dec;144(1-2):191-7.

[38] Weisberg LA. Thalamic hemorrhage: clinical-CT correlations. Neurology. 1986 Oct;36(10):1382-6.

[39] Walshe TM, Davis KR, Fisher CM. Thalamic hemorrhage: a computed tomographic-clinical correlation. Neurology. 1977 Mar;27(3):217-22.

[40] Barraquer-Bordas L, Illa I, Escartin A, Ruscalleda J, Marti-Vilalta JL. Thalamic hemorrhage. A study of 23 patients with diagnosis by computed tomography. Stroke J Cereb Circ. 1981 Aug;12(4):524-7.

[41] Kumral E, Kocaer T, Ertübey NO, Kumral K. Thalamic hemorrhage. A prospective study of 100 patients. Stroke J Cereb Circ. 1995 Jun;26(6):964-70.

[42] Ott KH, Kase CS, Ojemann RG, Mohr JP. Cerebellar hemorrhage: diagnosis and treatment. A review of 56 cases. Arch Neurol. 1974 Sep;31(3):160-7.

[43] Donauer E, Loew F, Faubert C, Alesch F, Schaan M. Prognostic factors in the treatment of cerebellar haemorrhage. Acta Neurochir (Wien). 1994;131(1-2):59-66.

[44] Kleinman JT, Hillis AE, Jordan LC. ABC/2: estimating intracerebral haemorrhage volume and total brain volume and predicting outcome in children. Dev Med Child Neurol. 2011 Mar;53(3):281-4.

[45] Safatlı DA, Günther A, Schlattmann P, Schwarz F, Kalff R, Ewald C. Predictors of 30-day mortality in patients with spontaneous primary intracerebral hemorrhage. Surg Neurol Int. 2016;7(Suppl 18):S510–S517.

[46] Linfante I, Llinas RH, Caplan LR, Warach S. MRI features of intracerebral hemorrhage within 2 hours from symptom onset. Stroke J Cereb Circ. 1999 Nov;30(11):2263-7.

[47] Mayer SA. Ultra-early hemostatic therapy for primary intracerebral hemorrhage: a review. Can J Neurol Sci J Can Sci Neurol. 2005 Dec;32(Suppl 2):S31–S37.

[48] Fujii Y, Takeuchi S, Sasaki O, Minakawa T, Tanaka R. Multivariate analysis of predictors of hematoma enlargement in spontaneous intracerebral hemorrhage. Stroke J Cereb Circ. 1998 Jun;29(6):1160-6.

[49] Murai Y, Takagi R, Ikeda Y, Yamamoto Y, Teramoto A. Three-dimensional computerized tomography angiography in patients with hyperacute intracerebral hemorrhage. J Neurosurg. 1999 Sep;91(3):424-31.

[50] Park SY, Kong MH, Kim JH, Kang DS, Song KY, Huh SK. Role of "Spot Sign" on CT angiography to predict hematoma expansion in spontaneous intracerebral hemorrhage. J Korean Neurosurg Soc. 2010 Nov;48(5):399-405.

[51] Kim SH, Jung HH, Whang K, Kim JY, Pyen JS, Oh JW. Which emphasizing factors are most predictive of hematoma expansion in spot sign positive intracerebral hemorrhage? J Korean Neurosurg Soc. 2014 Aug;56(2):86-90.

[52] Mendelow AD, Gregson BA, Mitchell PM, Murray GD, Rowan EN, Gholkar AR. Surgical trial in lobar intracerebral haemorrhage (STICH II) Protocol. Trials. 2011 May 17;12:124.

[53] Broderick JP. The STICH trial: what does it tell us and where do we go from here? Stroke J Cereb Circ. 2005 Jul;36(7):1619-20.

[54] Anderson CS, Heeley E, Huang Y, Wang J, Stapf C, Delcourt C, et al. Rapid blood-pressure lowering in patients with acute intracerebral hemorrhage. N Engl J Med. 2013 Jun 20;368(25):2355-65.

[55] Staykov D, Wagner I, Volbers B, Huttner HB, Doerfler A, Schwab S, et al. Dose effect of intraventricular fibrinolysis in ventricular hemorrhage. Stroke J Cereb Circ. 2011 Jul;42(7):2061-4.

[56] Hemphill JC, Greenberg SM, Anderson CS, Becker K, Bendok BR, Cushman M, et al. Guidelines for the management of spontaneous intracerebral hemorrhage: a guideline for healthcare professionals from the American Heart Association/American Stroke Association. Stroke J Cereb Circ. 2015 Jul;46(7):2032-60.

[57] Duff TA, Ayeni S, Levin AB, Javid M. Nonsurgical management of spontaneous intracerebral hematoma. Neurosurgery. 1981 Oct;9(4):387-93.

[58] Kamel H, Navi BB, Nakagawa K, Hemphill JC, Ko NU. Hypertonic saline versus mannitol for the treatment of elevated intracranial pressure: a meta-analysis of randomized clinical trials. Crit Care Med. 2011 Mar;39(3):554-9.

[59] Mayer SA, Brun NC, Begtrup K, Broderick J, Davis S, Diringer MN, et al. Recombinant activated factor VII for acute intracerebral hemorrhage. N Engl J Med. 2005 Feb 24;352(8):777-85.

[60] Mayer SA, Brun NC, Begtrup K, Broderick J, Davis S, Diringer MN, et al. Efficacy and safety of recombinant activated factor VII for acute intracerebral hemorrhage. N Engl J Med. 2008 May 15;358(20):2127-37.

[61] Schwarz S, Häfner K, Aschoff A, Schwab S. Incidence and prognostic significance of fever following intracerebral hemorrhage. Neurology. 2000 Jan 25;54(2):354-61.

[62] Takagi K. Body temperature in acute stroke. Stroke J Cereb Circ. 2002 Sep;33(9):2154-5.

[63] Kollmar R, Staykov D, Dörfler A, Schellinger PD, Schwab S, Bardutzky J. Hypothermia reduces perihemorrhagic edema after intracerebral hemorrhage. Stroke J Cereb Circ. 2010 Aug;41(8):1684-9.

[64] Stead LG, Gilmore RM, Bellolio MF, Mishra S, Bhagra A, Vaidyanathan L, et al. Hyperglycemia as an independent predictor of worse outcome in non-diabetic patients presenting with acute ischemic stroke. Neurocrit Care. 2009;10(2):181-6.

[65] Passero S, Ciacci G, Ulivelli M. The influence of diabetes and hyperglycemia on clinical course after intracerebral hemorrhage. Neurology. 2003 Nov 25;61(10):1351-6.

[66] NICE-SUGAR Study Investigators, Finfer S, Chittock DR, Su SY-S, Blair D, Foster D, et al. Intensive versus conventional glucose control in critically ill patients. N Engl J Med. 2009 Mar 26;360(13):1283-97.

[67] Beghi E, D'Alessandro R, Beretta S, Consoli D, Crespi V, Delaj L, et al. Incidence and predictors of acute symptomatic seizures after stroke. Neurology. 2011 Nov 15;77(20):1785-93.

[68] De Herdt V, Dumont F, Hénon H, Derambure P, Vonck K, Leys D, et al. Early seizures in intracerebral hemorrhage: incidence, associated factors, and outcome. Neurology. 2011 Nov 15;77(20):1794-800.

[69] Bladin CF, Alexandrov AV, Bellavance A, Bornstein N, Chambers B, Coté R, et al. Seizures after stroke: a prospective multicenter study. Arch Neurol. 2000 Nov;57(11):1617-22.

[70] Passero S, Rocchi R, Rossi S, Ulivelli M, Vatti G. Seizures after spontaneous supratentorial intracerebral hemorrhage. Epilepsia. 2002 Oct;43(10):1175-80.

[71] Messé SR, Sansing LH, Cucchiara BL, Herman ST, Lyden PD, Kasner SE, et al. Prophylactic antiepileptic drug use is associated with poor outcome following ICH. Neurocrit Care. 2009;11(1):38-44.

[72] Naidech AM, Garg RK, Liebling S, Levasseur K, Macken MP, Schuele SU, et al. Anticonvulsant use and outcomes after intracerebral hemorrhage. Stroke J Cereb Circ. 2009 Dec;40(12):3810-5.

[73] Gilad R, Boaz M, Dabby R, Sadeh M, Lampl Y. Are post intracerebral hemorrhage seizures prevented by anti-epileptic treatment? Epilepsy Res. 2011 Aug;95(3):227-31.

[74] Sandhu R, Aronow WS, Rajdev A, Sukhija R, Amin H, D'aquila K, et al. Relation of cardiac troponin I levels with in-hospital mortality in patients with ischemic stroke, intracerebral hemorrhage, and subarachnoid hemorrhage. Am J Cardiol. 2008 Sep 1;102(5):632-4.

[75] Touzé E, Varenne O, Chatellier G, Peyrard S, Rothwell PM, Mas J-L. Risk of myocardial infarction and vascular death after transient ischemic attack and ischemic stroke: a systematic review and meta-analysis. Stroke J Cereb Circ. 2005 Dec;36(12):2748-55.

[76] Holbrook A, Schulman S, Witt DM, Vandvik PO, Fish J, Kovacs MJ, et al. Evidence-based management of anticoagulant therapy: antithrombotic therapy and prevention of thrombosis, 9th ed: American college of chest physicians evidence-based clinical practice guidelines. Chest. 2012 Feb;141(Suppl 2):e152S–84S.

[77] Morgan T, Awad I, Keyl P, Lane K, Hanley D. Preliminary report of the clot lysis evaluating accelerated resolution of intraventricular hemorrhage (clear-IVH) clinical trial. Acta Neurochir Suppl. 2008;105:217-20.

[78] Naff N, Williams M, Keyl PM, Tuhrim S, Bullock MR, Mayer S, et al. Low-dose rt-PA enhances clot resolution in brain hemorrhage: the intraventricular hemorrhage thrombolysis trial. Stroke J Cereb Circ. 2011 Nov;42(11):3009-16.

[79] Webb AJS, Ullman NL, Mann S, Muschelli J, Awad IA, Hanley DF. Resolution of intraventricular hemorrhage varies by ventricular region and dose of intraventricular thrombolytic: the clot lysis: evaluating accelerated resolution of IVH (clear IVH) program. Stroke J Cereb Circ. 2012 Jun;43(6):1666-8.

[80] Chen C-C, Liu C-L, Tung Y-N, Lee H-C, Chuang H-C, Lin S-Z, et al. Endoscopic surgery for intraventricular hemorrhage (IVH) caused by thalamic hemorrhage: comparisons of endoscopic surgery and external ventricular drainage (EVD) surgery. World Neurosurg. 2011 Feb;75(2):264-8.

[81] Prasad K, Mendelow AD, Gregson B. Surgery for primary supratentorial intracerebral haemorrhage. Cochrane Database Syst Rev. 2008;(4):CD000200.

[82] Wang WZ, Jiang B, Liu HM, Li D, Lu CZ, Zhao YD, et al. Minimally invasive craniopuncture therapy vs. conservative treatment for spontaneous intracerebral hemorrhage: results from a randomized clinical trial in China. Int J Stroke Off J Int Stroke Soc. 2009 Feb;4(1):11-6.

[83] Fung C, Murek M, Z'Graggen WJ, Krähenbühl AK, Gautschi OP, Schucht P, et al. Decompressive hemicraniectomy in patients with supratentorial intracerebral hemorrhage. Stroke J Cereb Circ. 2012 Dec;43(12):3207-11.

[84] Benes V, Vladyka V, Zvěrina E. Sterotaxic evacuation of typical brain haemorrhage. Acta Neurochir (Wien). 1965;13(3):419-26.

[85] Rabinstein AA, Tisch SH, McClelland RL, Wijdicks EFM. Cause is the main predictor of outcome in patients with pontine hemorrhage. Cerebrovasc Dis Basel Switz. 2004;17(1):66-71.

[86] Cohen ZR, Ram Z, Knoller N, Peles E, Hadani M. Management and outcome of non-traumatic cerebellar haemorrhage. Cerebrovasc Dis Basel Switz. 2002;14(3-4):207-13.

[87] van Loon J, Van Calenbergh F, Goffin J, Plets C. Controversies in the management of spontaneous cerebellar haemorrhage. A consecutive series of 49 cases and review of the literature. Acta Neurochir (Wien). 1993;122(3-4):187-93.

[88] Aghi M, Ogilvy C. Surgical Management of Intracerebral hemorrhage. In: Quinones-Hinojosa, editor. Schmidek & Sweet Operative Neurosurgical Techniques. 6th ed. Philadelphia: Elsevier/Saunders; 2012. pp. 823-36.

[89] Hemphill JC, Bonovich DC, Besmertis L, Manley GT, Johnston SC. The ICH score: a simple, reliable grading scale for intracerebral hemorrhage. Stroke J Cereb Circ. 2001 Apr;32(4):891-7.

Chapter 3

Surgical Management of Intracerebral Hemorrhage

Arvin R. Wali, Kevin Porras, Peter Abraham,
Michael G. Brandel, David Santiago Dieppa,
Jeffrey Steinberg, Scott Pannell and
Alexander A. Khalessi

Additional information is available at the end of the chapter

http://dx.doi.org/10.5772/67633

Abstract

Intracerebral hemorrhage (ICH), defined as bleeding within the brain parenchyma, remains a challenging and controversial neurosurgical entity to treat. ICH has a broad range of etiology—stemming from complications associated with traumatic head injury to complications of hemorrhagic stroke. The role of medical management lies in optimizing blood pressure and intracerebral pressure, preventing secondary injury from complications of the hematoma such as seizures, and correcting coagulopathy. Given the mass effect of a hematoma and the possibility of expansion, surgical interventions attempt to evacuate the clot to restore normal intracerebral pressure and prevent worsening neurologic injury. This chapter reviews the recent controversy associated with surgical evacuation of intracerebral hemorrhage placing particular emphasis on the size and location of the hemorrhage and the methods used to evacuate the expanding ICH. Moreover, this chapter reviews considerations and therapeutic goals of the preoperative and postoperative window to minimize complications and optimize patient care.

Keywords: intracerebral hemorrhage, hemorrhagic stroke, surgical intracerebral hemorrhage, neurosurgical interventions

1. Introduction

Intracerebral hemorrhage (ICH) is defined as bleeding that takes place within the brain parenchyma and impacts 63,000 people annually within the United States [1, 2]. ICH is a major complication of traumatic brain injury and contributes to 15% of strokes [3]. Many etiologies are implicated in ICH, including hypertension, vascular anomalies, amyloid angiopathy, coagulopathy, brain malignancies, pregnancies, and substance abuse. Depending on the extent of hemorrhage and additional risk factors, ICH prognosis can be highly variable. Extensive hemorrhage has been associated with greater than 30% mortality rate within one month of injury with only 30% of patients returning to independent functioning by 6 months [4].

Medical management aims to optimize blood pressure, intracerebral pressure (ICP), coagulopathy, seizure control, fever control, and deep vein thrombosis prophylaxis. Additionally, surgical management aims to prevent neurologic decline through surgical decompression of the skull and evacuation of expanding hematoma [5]. However, the role of surgery in management for ICH remains controversial, and numerous trials have been conducted examining the indications and efficacy of prompt surgical intervention. This chapter will explore the current scientific literature regarding the indications and efficacy of neurosurgical intervention in the management of patients with ICH.

2. Preoperative diagnostics and workup

ICH presents with acute-onset focal neurologic deficits, headache (approximately 40% of patients), elevated systolic blood pressure (50%), nausea, and vomiting (50%) [5–7]. Common deficits include, in order of decreasing incidence, paresis, sensory deficits, speech deficits, vision changes, and gait disturbances [6]. Symptoms are often progressive due to hematoma expansion, which tends to occur within the first several hours following ICH. However, patients without hemorrhage growth may still experience substantial neurological deterioration within the first 24 hours [8]. Electrographic seizures may occur in up to a third of patients with ICH, although only half of these are clinically significant [9]. Seizures are more likely to occur with cortical involvement of ICH and may be associated with neurological deterioration and increased midline shift [10, 11]. Patients commonly have altered mental status, and those with large or growing hematomas may experience rapid worsening in Glasgow Coma Scale (GCS) [12].

Non-contrast computed tomography (CT) scan is considered to be the "gold standard" for diagnosis of new ICH and detection of other forms of intracranial bleeding that may present concomitantly [13]. Magnetic resonance imaging (MRI) may also be beneficial in identifying microhemorrhages, and CT angiogram is sensitive in identifying secondary causes of intraparenchymal bleeding such as aneurysm rupture, vasculitis, intracranial malignancy, or arteriovenous malformations [14, 15].

In an emergency setting, ensuring adequate airway, breathing, and cerebral perfusion is essential. For patients with a GCS < 8, transtentorial herniation, intraventricular hemorrhage, or hydrocephalus, an ICP monitor should be placed to dynamically monitor cerebral perfusion pressure [16]. Management of elevated ICPs in the acute setting includes elevating the head of bed to 30°, sedation, intubation, and hyperventilation of the patient to a $PaCO_2$ of 25–30 and rapidly infusing hypertonic saline or mannitol while preparing the operating room for surgical decompression or clot evacuation [9, 17]. Management of hemorrhagic mass effect and acute hydrocephalus via external ventricular drain is beneficial for ICP measurement and cerebrospinal fluid (CSF) diversion in these patients and has been shown to significantly reduce mortality in the setting of intraventricular hemorrhage [18, 19].

3. Surgical management

The role of surgery in the treatment of intracerebral hemorrhage remains a matter of debate. Though many clinical trials have attempted to better characterize the role of surgical evacuation in ICH, variability in factors such as location and volume of the bleed and method of surgical intervention have long limited extrapolation to guidelines. Much less controversy surrounds the surgical management of infratentorial ICH due to proximity to the brain stem and the possibility of catastrophic injury and complications [20, 21]. For this reason, posterior fossa hematomas greater than 3 cm are evacuated due to the significant risk of brain stem compression and hydrocephalus [22].

Regardless of the cause of ICH, close monitoring of complications such as hypertension, hematoma expansion, perihematomal edema, seizures, intraventricular hemorrhage leading to hydrocephalus, and venous thromboembolism is vital to patient survival and prevention of functional deficits [23]. In addition to reducing intracranial pressure, surgical evacuation reduces clot volume, which contributes to both mechanical compression of the brain and neurotoxic edema [24]. Despite these perceived benefits, clinical trials prior to 2004 failed to demonstrate a clear survival difference in patients offered surgical intervention and medical treatment compared to conservative medical management. For example, a multicenter randomized controlled trial utilizing minimally invasive, stereotactic approaches with low-dose tissue plasminogen activator (tPA) for liquefaction and aspiration of clot (SICHPA trial) demonstrated effective reduction of clot size compared to conservative treatment, but no differences were found in 180-day mortality rates [25].

Five trials from 1989 to 2003 demonstrated equivocal outcomes following surgical intervention. Encouraging functional outcomes were demonstrated in a small study of stereotactic evacuation of putaminal hemorrhages in 2004 [26]. The International Surgical Trial in Intracerebral Hemorrhage (STICH) randomized over 1000 patients with spontaneous basal ganglia and/or lobar hemorrhages to surgery within 24 hours of presentation versus early conservative management with possible surgical evacuation after 24 hours in the setting of neurological deterioration to examine the efficacy of early surgical clot evacuation. Though the trial found only 26% of surgical patients had favorable outcomes at 6 months compared to 24% in the medical management group, subgroup analysis demonstrated that patients with supratentorial ICH with hematomas 1 cm or less from the cortical surface had improved outcomes with surgical evacuation compared with patients with deep hematomas and conservative management [27].

To follow up on this finding, over 600 patients with 10–100 mL superficial lobar hemorrhages and no intraventricular hemorrhage (IVH) were randomized to evacuation within 12 hours plus medical treatment compared to medical management alone with the option for subsequent surgical intervention for neurological deterioration in the STICH II trial in 2013 [28]. This trial demonstrated similarly statistically insignificant findings. Mortality at 6 months was 18% in the early surgery group compared to 24% in the medical management group, with an absolute difference of 5.6%. Though the surgery group demonstrated no vegetative survivors through 6 months and the distribution of Extended Glasgow Outcome Scale (GOS-E) scores was more favorable in the surgery group, neither of these findings was statistically significant. However, subgroup analysis of patients with poor prognosis before treatment defined as GCS 9–12 demonstrated more favorable outcome with surgery (odds ratio of poor outcome: 0.49, 95% confidence interval 0.26–0.92, p = 0.02). Based upon the results of the STICH II trial, the investigators concluded that patients with higher GCS of 13–15 do not demonstrate survival advantage with early surgery if given the option of delayed surgery if deterioration occurs.

The CLEAR IVH trial and MISTIE trial are ongoing investigations that use minimally invasive technique with assistance of low-dose tPA [29]. Preliminary results from the MISTIE II trial demonstrated minimally invasive aspiration with low-dose tPA reduced clots to 50% of the stabilized volume within the first week, compared to a 6% reduction with medical management alone. Though statistically significant increases in symptomatic bleeding were not seen with the use of tPA (2.4% in the minimally invasive plus tPA group versus 9.3% in the medical management group), the authors did caution that the use of minimally invasive techniques with tPA did increase asymptomatic hemorrhages (22.2% versus 7.1%, p = 0.051). These results demonstrate the safety and efficacy of these interventions compared with conservative management alone [30]. Furthermore, hematoma evacuation has been shown to significantly reduce perihematomal edema, even when combined with tPA delivered to the clot [31]. The MISTIE Intraoperative Stereotactic Computed Tomography-Guided Endoscopic Surgery (MISTIE ICES) trial [32] was recently completed and demonstrated 42.9% of surgical patients had functional neurological outcomes defined as a modified Rankin scale score (mRS) of 0–3, compared to 23.7% in the medical management group at 180 and 365 days (p = 0.19). These results demonstrate the safety and efficacy of CT-guided endoscopic surgery to remove acute ICH. Examples of endoscopic hemorrhage evacuation can be found below (**Figures 1–3**).

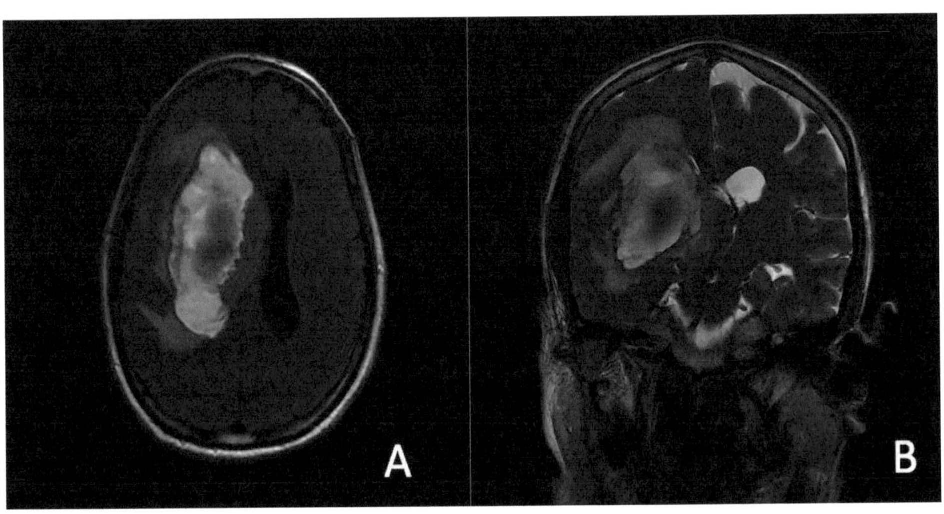

Figure 1. (A and B): Axial and coronal MRI demonstrating right-sided preoperative intracerebral hemorrhage involving the right ventricle.

http://dx.doi.org/10.5772/67633

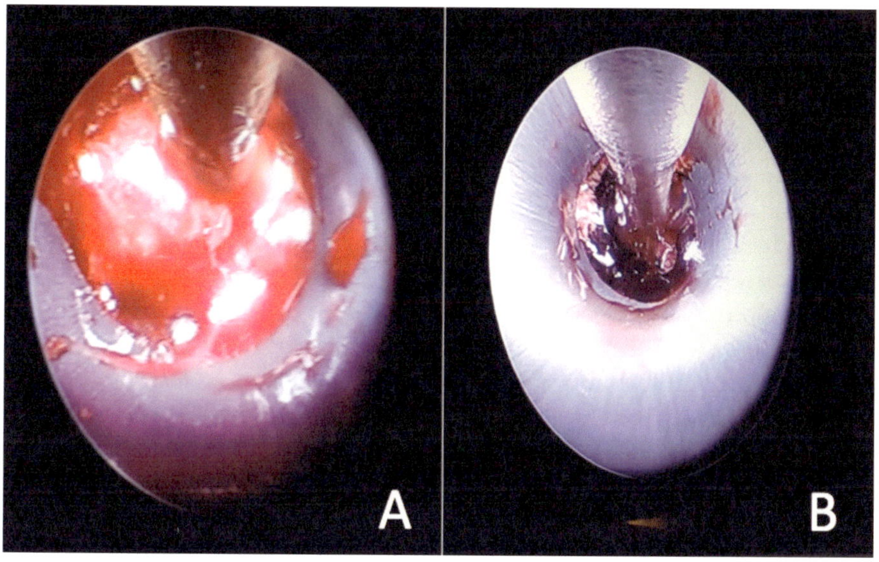

Figure 2. (A and B): Intraoperative endoscopic clot evacuation using minimally invasive technique.

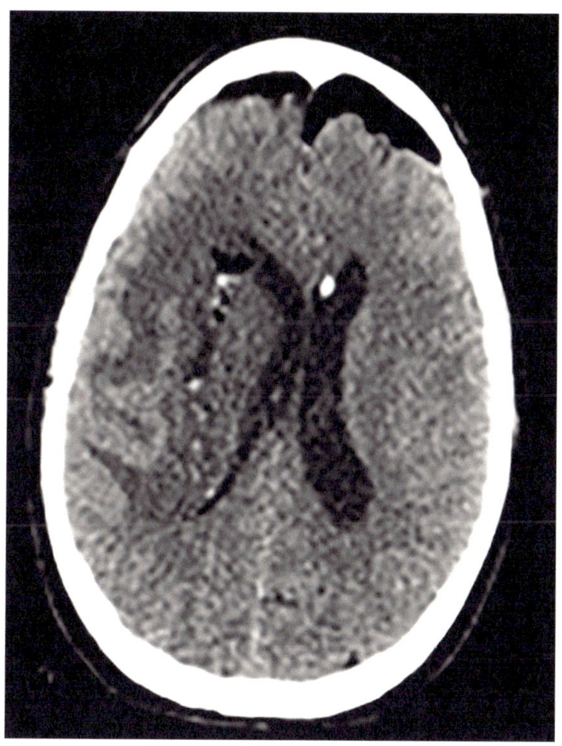

Figure 3. Follow-up axial CT scan after endoscopic hemorrhagic evacuation demonstrating resolution of clot.

4. Endoscopic hemorrhage evacuation example

Taken together, the results of these trials demonstrate the difficulties in producing guidelines for the surgical management of ICH (**Figures 1–3**). Though surgical intervention demonstrates better outcomes in early trials, these findings do not reach statistical significance. Like many neurosurgical studies, many of these trials suffer from significant patient crossover and highly variable patient characteristics. It has been argued that the subjectively better outcomes in early trials are of clinical relevance, especially when patients are projected to have poor outcomes as a result of the location or volume of their bleed. More recent trials have demonstrated the safety and efficacy of endoscopic measures combined with low-dose tPA in dissolving clots, reducing edema, and improving outcomes to a statistically significant degree. Endoscopic approaches to ICH will likely become more widely utilized as more data from clinical trials becomes available.

5. Postoperative management

Postoperative management of ICH includes ensuring appropriate blood pressure control, frequent neurologic examinations, deep vein thrombosis prophylaxis, and gastric ulcer prophylaxis. Subsequent physical therapy and rehabilitation especially in the first month after ICH has been shown to be more effective in increasing independence with activities of daily life and motor function when compared to controls [33].

Despite limited evidence of long-term postoperative management of ICH, studies suggest that ICH patients would benefit from a systolic blood pressure of <130 mmHg. Patients, notably, with established small vessel disease see a 60% risk reduction in recurrent ICH with these blood pressure guidelines [9]. Furthermore, studies have shown that in patients with poor clinical grade or coexisting cardiopulmonary complications, early hemodynamic stabilization is associated with lower rates of delayed cerebral ischemia, lower 90-day mRS, and lower length of intensive care unit stay [34].

Deep vein thrombosis (DVT) prophylaxis after ICH is a current area of uncertainty. Various studies, including the CLOTS3 trial, show reduction in asymptomatic DVT with the use of intermittent pneumatic compression devices in ICH patients. Similarly, low molecular weight heparin or unfractionated heparin can be used for DVT prophylaxis in patients with stable hematomas or 24 hours after craniotomy [35]. There is little current evidence to suggest positive or negative outcomes of mortality with gastric ulcer prophylaxis for ICH patients. A randomized controlled trial comparing ranitidine, sucralfate, and placebo for gastric hemorrhage prophylaxis in ICH patients showed no significant difference in mortality or pneumonia. However, given the increased prevalence of gastric ulcers in these patients, prophylaxis should be initiated based on current data [36].

6. Conclusion

Intracerebral hemorrhage remains a serious complication associated with head trauma and a consequence of hemorrhagic stroke. Appropriate diagnosis and management of intracerebral pressures and ventilation preoperatively remains an important opportunity to improve patient outcomes. While surgical intervention for large infratentorial ICH is clearly beneficial, the role of supratentorial ICH remains controversial given the diversity of ICH locations, depth of bleed, and technique used to evacuate the hemorrhagic clot. Superficial cortical ICH can have improved outcomes with surgical evacuation compared to medical management alone, and image-guided endoscopic evacuation of clot also shows promise. ICH patients can have a host of complications in the postoperative window and require close follow-up to prevent subsequent surgical and medical complications. Further prospective trials elucidating whether surgical intervention compared to medical management alone is optimal given an ICH location, presentation, or volume of hemorrhage will continue to guide the management of this diverse population.

Author details

Arvin R. Wali, Kevin Porras, Peter Abraham, Michael G. Brandel, David Santiago Dieppa, Jeffrey Steinberg, Scott Pannell and Alexander A. Khalessi*

*Address all correspondence to: akhalessi@ucsd.edu

Department of Neurosurgery, University of California, San Diego, La Jolla, California, USA

References

[1] Rincon F, Mayer SA. The epidemiology of intracerebral hemorrhage in the United States from 1979 to 2008. Neurocrit Care 2013;19(1):95-102.

[2] Sahni R, Weinberger J. Management of intracerebral hemorrhage. Vasc Health Risk Manag 2007;3(5):701-709.

[3] Perel P, Roberts I, Bouamra O, Woodford M, Mooney J, Lecky F. Intracranial bleeding in patients with traumatic brain injury: a prognostic study. BMC Emerg Med 2009;9:15.

[4] Greenberg MS Handbook of Neurosurgery. 8th edition. ed. New York: Thieme; 2016.

[5] Broderick JP, Adams HP, Jr., Barsan W, et al. Guidelines for the management of spontaneous intracerebral hemorrhage: A statement for healthcare professionals from a special writing group of the stroke council, American heart association. Stroke 1999;30(4):905-915.

[6] Rathore SS, Hinn AR, Cooper LS, Tyroler HA, Rosamond WD. Characterization of incident stroke signs and symptoms: Findings from the atherosclerosis risk in communities study. Stroke 2002;33(11):2718-2721.

[7] Dandapani BK, Suzuki S, Kelley RE, Reyes-Iglesias Y, Duncan RC. Relation between blood pressure and outcome in intracerebral hemorrhage. Stroke 1995;26(1):21-24.

[8] Brott T, Broderick J, Kothari R, et al. Early hemorrhage growth in patients with intracerebral hemorrhage. Stroke 1997;28(1):1-5.

[9] Hemphill JC, 3rd, Greenberg SM, Anderson CS, et al. Guidelines for the management of spontaneous intracerebral hemorrhage: A guideline for healthcare professionals from the American heart association/American stroke association. Stroke 2015;46(7):2032-2060.

[10] Vespa PM, O'Phelan K, Shah M, et al. Acute seizures after intracerebral hemorrhage: A factor in progressive midline shift and outcome. Neurology 2003;60(9):1441-1446.

[11] Bladin CF, Alexandrov AV, Bellavance A, et al. Seizures after stroke: A prospective multicenter study. Arch Neurol 2000;57(11):1617-1622.

[12] Radberg JA, Olsson JE, Radberg CT. Prognostic parameters in spontaneous intracerebral hematomas with special reference to anticoagulant treatment. Stroke 1991;22(5):571-576.

[13] Fiebach JB, Schellinger PD, Gass A, et al. Stroke magnetic resonance imaging is accurate in hyperacute intracerebral hemorrhage: A multicenter study on the validity of stroke imaging. Stroke 2004;35(2):502-506.

[14] Kidwell CS, Saver JL, Villablanca JP, et al. Magnetic resonance imaging detection of microbleeds before thrombolysis: An emerging application. Stroke 2002;33(1):95-98.

[15] Nentwich LM, Veloz W. Neuroimaging in acute stroke. Emerg Med Clin North Am 2012;30(3):659-680.

[16] Goldstein JN, Gilson AJ. Critical care management of acute intracerebral hemorrhage. Curr Treat Options Neurol 2011;13(2):204-216.

[17] Mirsen T. Acute treatment of hypertensive intracerebral hemorrhage. Curr Treat Options Neurol 2010;12(6):504-517.

[18] Dey M, Jaffe J, Stadnik A, Awad IA. External ventricular drainage for intraventricular hemorrhage. Curr Neurol Neurosci Rep 2012;12(1):24-33.

[19] Lovasik BP, McCracken DJ, McCracken CE, et al. The effect of external ventricular drain use in intracerebral hemorrhage. World Neurosurg 2016;94:309-318.

[20] Poon MT, Fonville AF, Al-Shahi Salman R. Long-term prognosis after intracerebral haemorrhage: Systematic review and meta-analysis. J Neurol Neurosurg Psychiatry 2014;85(6):660-667.

[21] Hemphill JC, 3rd, Bonovich DC, Besmertis L, Manley GT, Johnston SC. The ICH score: A simple, reliable grading scale for intracerebral hemorrhage. Stroke 2001;32(4):891-897.

[22] Morgenstern L, Hemphill 3rd J, Anderson C, et al. American Heart Association Stroke Council and Council on Cardiovascular Nursing. Guidelines for the management of spontaneous intracerebral hemorrhage: a guideline for healthcare professionals from the American Heart Association/American Stroke Association. Stroke; a journal of cerebral circulation. 2010;41(9):2108-2129.

[23] Rennert RC, Signorelli JW, Abraham P, Pannell JS, Khalessi AA. Minimally invasive treatment of intracerebral hemorrhage. Expert Rev Neurother 2015;15(8):919-933.

[24] RF, et al. Role of blood clot formation on early edema development after experimental intracerebral hemorrhage. Stroke; a journal of cerebral circulation. 1998;29(12):2580-2586.

[25] Teernstra OP, Evers SM, Lodder J, Leffers P, Franke CL, Blaauw G. Stereotactic treatment of intracerebral hematoma by means of a plasminogen activator: A multicenter randomized controlled trial (SICHPA). Stroke 2003;34(4):968-974.

[26] Hattori N, Katayama Y, Maya Y, Gatherer A. Impact of stereotactic hematoma evacuation on activities of daily living during the chronic period following spontaneous putaminal hemorrhage: a randomized study. J Neurosurg. 2004;101(3):417-420.

[27] Mendelow AD, Gregson BA, Fernandes HM, et al. Early surgery versus initial conservative treatment in patients with spontaneous supratentorial intracerebral haematomas in the international surgical trial in intracerebral haemorrhage (STICH): A randomised trial. Lancet 2005;365(9457):387-397.

[28] Mendelow AD, Gregson BA, Rowan EN, Murray GD, Gholkar A, Mitchell PM. Early surgery versus initial conservative treatment in patients with spontaneous supratentorial lobar intracerebral haematomas (STICH II): A randomised trial. Lancet 2013;382(9890):397-408.

[29] Dey M, Stadnik A, Awad IA. Spontaneous intracerebral and intraventricular hemorrhage: advances in minimally invasive surgery and thrombolytic evacuation, and lessons learned in recent trials. Neurosurgery 2014;74(Suppl 1):S142–S150.

[30] Hanley DF, Thompson RE, Muschelli J, et al. Safety and efficacy of minimally invasive surgery plus alteplase in intracerebral haemorrhage evacuation (MISTIE): A randomised, controlled, open-label, phase 2 trial. Lancet Neurol 2016;15(12):1228-1237.

[31] Mould WA, Carhuapoma JR, Muschelli J, et al. Minimally invasive surgery plus recombinant tissue-type plasminogen activator for intracerebral hemorrhage evacuation decreases perihematomal edema. Stroke 2013;44(3):627-634.

[32] Vespa P, Hanley D, Betz J, et al. ICES (intraoperative stereotactic computed tomography-guided endoscopic surgery) for brain hemorrhage: A multicenter randomized controlled trial. Stroke 2016;47(11):2749-2755.

[33] Bai Y, Hu Y, Wu Y, et al. A prospective, randomized, single-blinded trial on the effect of early rehabilitation on daily activities and motor function of patients with hemorrhagic stroke. J Clin Neurosci 2012;19(10):1376-1379.

[34] Mutoh T, Kazumata K, Terasaka S, Taki Y, Suzuki A, Ishikawa T. Early intensive versus minimally invasive approach to postoperative hemodynamic management after subarachnoid hemorrhage. Stroke 2014;45(5):1280-1284.

[35] Nyquist P, Bautista C, Jichici D, et al. Prophylaxis of venous thrombosis in neurocritical care patients: An evidence-based guideline: A statement for healthcare professionals from the neurocritical care society. Neurocrit Care 2016;24(1):47-60.

[36] Misra UK, Kalita J, Pandey S, Mandal SK, Srivastava M. A randomized placebo controlled trial of ranitidine versus sucralfate in patients with spontaneous intracerebral hemorrhage for prevention of gastric hemorrhage. J Neurol Sci 2005;239(1):5-10.

Chapter 4

Neuroimaging in Intracerebral Hemorrhage

Shazia Mirza and Sankalp Gokhale

Additional information is available at the end of the chapter

http://dx.doi.org/10.5772/67303

Abstract

Hemorrhagic stroke accounts for 15% of all strokes but results in nearly a third of the mortality. Neuroimaging forms the mainstay in diagnosis, which has resulted in improved treatment outcomes. The mandate of neuroimaging includes management, risk assessment, prognostication, and research. This involves rapid identification not only to direct treatment but also to discover the underlying etiology such as vascular malformations or tumors, monitor the evolving course of the hemorrhage and rapidly identify complications. While computed tomography (CT) remains the imaging of choice to rapidly detect acute hemorrhage, growing evidence shows that magnetic resonance imaging (MRI) is comparable to CT for detecting blood in the immediate setting and superior in this regard at subacute and chronic time points. Several advances have been made in the image sequencing protocols to detect bleeds at varying time points and to distinguish possible etiology. Initial and serial imaging is used to identify patients who may benefit from intervention. Advances in this field such as diffusion tensor imaging and functional MRI are being studied for their impact in understanding the extent of injury and possible recovery mechanisms, possibly allowing prognostication for patients.

Keywords: intracerebral hemorrhage, hemorrhagic strokes, neuroimaging, computed tomography, magnetic resonance imaging, vascular malformations

1. Introduction

Hemorrhagic stroke is responsible for 15% of all strokes occurring annually in the United States and has a high mortality rate of 29% [1]. About two-thirds of these strokes are intracerebral hemorrhage (ICH) and one-third are subarachnoid hemorrhage (SAH) for which neuroimaging forms the mainstay in diagnosis; as history, clinical symptoms and signs are often nonspecific but have resulted in improved treatment outcomes.

2. Definitions

Intracranial hemorrhage is the accumulation of blood within the skull, the parenchyma and/or the meningeal spaces and/or other associated potential spaces (epidural and subdural). The term intracerebral hemorrhage refers to bleeding in the brain parenchyma (white or gray matter). The term subarachnoid hemorrhage is used for blood collection in the subarachnoid space (i.e., in the space between the pia and arachnoid meningeal layers). ICH is classified conventionally as primary or secondary, based on its causes, with primary ICH (80–85% of ICH) related to hypertension and amyloid angiopathy and secondary ICH having varied etiologies such as drugs, malformations, tumors, vasculitis, etc. [2]. This has given way to different systems of classification such as SMASH-U and lobar vs. deep.

Our chapter aims to:

- Explain the various modalities which can be used in the detection of ICH with a brief description of their mechanism.
- Provide advantages and disadvantages of each method.
- Provide image descriptions of common findings in ICH with sample images.
- Explain the modalities used in Detecting the etiology of ICH and complications with image findings.
- List some common sequences in practice today.
- Explain the expanded role of imaging from management to prognostication.

The goals of neuroimaging include:

The main goal of neuroimaging in a patient with suspected cerebral hemorrhage is to find a modality with perfect sensitivity and specificity. Rapid and accurate identification of hemorrhage is critical in planning therapy.

- Detecting intracerebral hemorrhage (ICH).
- Detecting etiology.
- Detecting tissue at risk.
- Detecting complications such as vasospasm, mass effect, and herniation.
- Detecting hemorrhagic complications in ischemic infarcts.
- Assessing risk factors for hemorrhage.
- Detecting resolution—monitoring and management.
- Prognostication of recovery.
- Assisting in research endeavors to advance both knowledge and treatment in ICH patients.

3. Early detection

3.1. Need

ICH is a medical Emergency, with rapid diagnosis and management being vital due to early and rapid hematoma expansion and clinical deterioration. This increases the mortality to as high as 75% in patients with pre-hospital neurological decline and results in worsened long term outcomes [3]. Since clinical features such as severe headache, high blood pressure, vomiting, loss of consciousness, and rapid progression cannot always be relied upon as being specific for hemorrhagic stroke, neuroimaging is mandatory.

3.2. Protocol

Rapid neuroimaging with noncontrast computed tomography (NCCT) or magnetic resonance imaging (MRI) is recommended to distinguish ischemic stroke from ICH [3]. Noncontrast CT (NCCT), perfusion CT, and CT angiography (CTA) are usually used in the hyperacute stroke setting. The imaging appearance of the ICH is closely linked to the physiological processes at play during and after the bleeding event.

4. ICH appearance on CT

4.1. NCCT

Bleeding into the cerebral parenchyma results in a hematoma consisting of proteins, serum, platelets, white blood cells, and red blood cells (with hemoglobin), and the concentration of the latter (relative to plasma) is responsible for the degree of attenuation of the X-ray beam. The varied components of the hematoma give it a heterogeneous appearance. The attenuation of blood with a normal hematocrit (45%) is much higher (56 Hounsfield units—HU) than gray matter (37–41 HU) and white matter (30–24 HU) resulting in the 'brighter' or 'whiter' region in patients with a normal hematocrit [4] (**Table 1**, **Figure 1**).

At the immediate onset of the bleed, (hyperacute phase) the blood has a similar attenuation as that of the cortex and is hard to distinguish. However, within minutes after a clot forms (platelet clumps, and proteins are consumed), the degree of attenuation increases and continues to increase over the hours as the clot retracts and extrudes serum, seen markedly in the center of the hematoma.

Within hours, the hematoma is surrounded by vasogenic edema which may last up to 2 weeks. Vasogenic edema is the extravasation of fluid and proteins into the extracellular spaces, due to the loss of integrity of the blood brain barrier and hence has a hypoattenuated or "darker" appearance on CT scan images, surrounding the hematoma.

In a large bleed, a fluid level may be visualized on imaging within hours of onset as the cellular debris collects in the more gravity-dependent portion, giving that area a higher attenuation.

Time	Process	CT
Immediately on extravasation	Bleeding into parenchyma	Hyperattenuated (brighter) lesion Heterogeneous due to varied cellular components
Minutes	Clot formation, serum extruded	Increasing intensity, marked in the center of hematoma
Hours–2 weeks	Vasogenic edema surrounds bleed	Hypoattenuated or "darker" appearance on CT scan images, surrounding the hematoma
Hours	Cellular debris settles in the gravity dependent part	Fluid level (with hyperattenuated dependent portion)
Days–weeks	Clot breakdown by scavengers (macrophages)	Decrease in attenuation beginning at periphery toward the center
2–3 weeks	Resolution of clot	Same intensity as white matter
Weeks-months	Cavity: collapsed or filled with cerebrospinal fluid	Small slit like cavity which may or may not be visualized
Months	Encephalomalacia	Hypointense (darker) area at lesion site

Table 1. CT imaging of intracerebral hemorrhage.

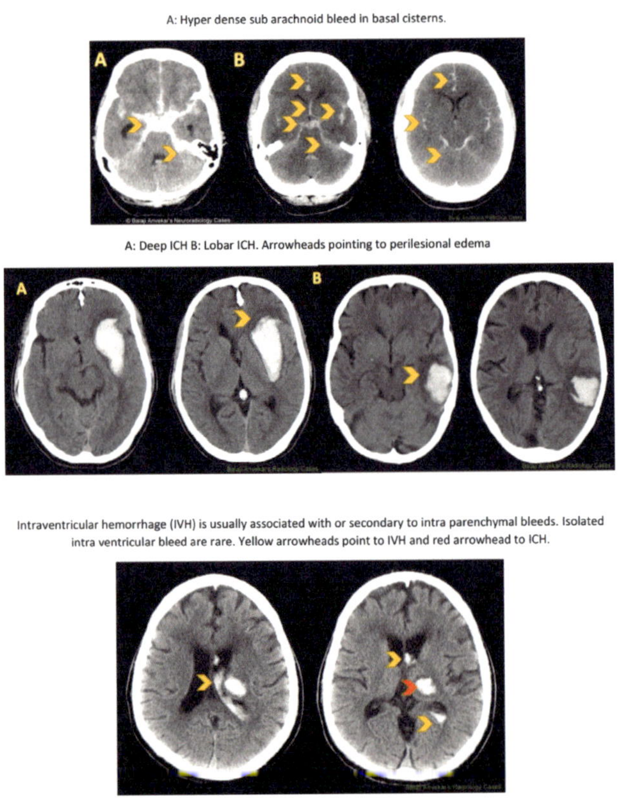

Figure 1. Immediate detection of hemorrhage using NCCT: the first image has yellow arrowheads pointing to hyperdense areas representing sub-arachnoid bleeding in the basal cisterns. The second image has yellow arrowheads pointing to peri lesional edema around deep ICH (A) and lobar ICH (B). The third image shows Intraventricular hemorrhage (IVH) (yellow arrowhead) which is usually associated with or secondary to intra parenchymal bleeds (red arrowhead).

The breakdown of the clot by natural scavengers such as macrophages continues over several days and results in a decrease in attenuation beginning at the periphery and working its way toward the center, gradually over a period of 4–9 days having the same attenuation as cortical gray matter and eventually after 2–3 weeks, having a similar attenuation as white matter.

This explains the difficulty in using CT scan to detect subacute hemorrhages due to similar appearance (iso-attenuation) with the parenchyma, and it is often scarce or difficult to distinguish mass effect and edema, which is fortunately obviated by the use of MRI.

The hematoma is eventually resolved into a small or slit like fluid filled cavity which may or may not be appreciated on CT scan. Eventually the only evidence of the hemorrhage may be encephalomalacia (hypointense or 'darker' appearance) at the location.

The use of contrast material with CT scan, usually performed nonemergently for reasons other than initial detection does not usually show enhancement although it may develop after weeks or months at the periphery of the resolving hematoma, which may make it hard to distinguish it from tumors or abscesses [5].

4.2. CT angiography (CTA)

Contrast extravasation within the hematoma is used to identify patients at risk for hematoma expansion, which is commonly referred to as the "Spot Sign," which is used as a predictor of poor neurological outcomes. This can be used to institute prothrombotic therapies such as Factor VII and increased surveillance to avoid poor outcomes. CTA performed within 96 hours of the event has >95% sensitivity and specificity in identifying vascular malformations. However, this must be balanced with the severe contrast associated complications such as allergy and nephropathy as well as possible effects on the blood brain barrier.

4.3. Quantification

NCCT is used to quantify hematoma volume and monitor its evolution. ICH volume is calculated using the ABC/2 method. A = greatest hemorrhage diameter, B = diameter at 90° to A, and C = approximate number of CT slices with hemorrhage multiplied by slice thickness. This method however has been shown to have a large margin of error especially for irregularly shaped bleeds (by an excess of 7.33 cm^3 when compared to manual planimetric method [6].

5. ICH appearance on MRI

The MRI appearance of ICH is based on the evolution of the hematoma over time (as explained above for CT) and the corresponding signal characteristics. The MR signal characteristics in turn are dependent mainly on the chemical state of the iron molecules in hemoglobin as well as the state of the red blood cell membrane (**Table 2**, **Figure 2**).

Time	Process	State of iron	State of membrane	T1 effect	T2 effect	T1 weighted images	T2 weighted images
Hyperacute							
Immediate -hours	Bleeding into parenchyma	Oxygenated (diamagnetic iron)	Intact	none	No susceptibility effect	Hypo- or isointense	Mildly hyper- or iso intense
	Deoxygenation at periphery begins	Deoxygenated at periphery (paramagnetic iron)	Intact	None	Susceptibility effect +	No change	Hypointense rim at periphery
Acute							
Hours–days	Deoxygenation from the outside in	Deoxygenated (paramagnetic iron)	Intact	None	Susceptibility effect +	Hypo- or isointense	Hypointense lesion
	Oxidation of iron at periphery	Met-hemoglobin at periphery	Intact	Decrease in T1 relaxation	None	Mild hyperintensity at periphery	None
Early subacute							
Days-weeks (usually 1 week)	Oxidation of iron to ferric state	Met-hemoglobin	Intact	Decrease in T1 relaxation	Susceptibility effect +	Hyperintense lesion	Hypointense lesion
Late subacute							
Week-months	Oxidation of iron to ferric state	Met-hemoglobin	Degraded	Decrease in T1 relaxation	No susceptibility effect	Hyperintense lesion	Hyperintense lesion
Chronic							
Several months	Protein breakdown	By-products	Degraded	Reduced signal intensity	Reduced signal intensity	Decreased hyperintensity	Decreased hyperintensity
	Iron deposited as hemosiderin at rim	Hemosiderin	Compartmentalized in molecule	None	Susceptibility effect +	Isoattenuation.	Hypointense rim
	CSF-filled cavity or slit-like cavity	—	—			Hypointense fluid-filled or slit-like cavity	Hyperintense fluid-filled or slit-like cavity

• CSF = cerebrospinal fluid.

Table 2. MR imaging of intracerebral hemorrhage.

http://dx.doi.org/10.5772/67303

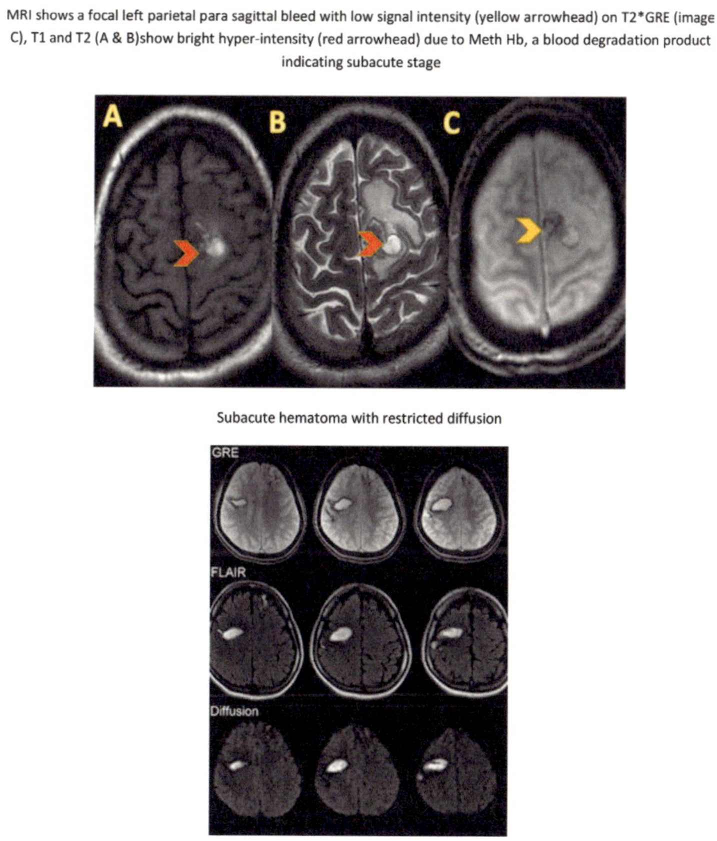

Figure 2. MR appearance of ICH: (Top) MRI shows a focal left parietal para sagittal bleed with low signal intensity (yellow arrowhead) on T2*GRE (image C), T1 and T2 (A & B) show a bright hyper-intensity (red arrowhead) due to Meth Hb, a blood degradation product indicating a sub-acute bleed. (Bottom) MRI showing sub-acute hematoma with restricted diffusion.

Iron within an intact red cell membrane causes shortened T2 relaxation times known as Susceptibility effect (which is lost when the membrane degrades and the hemoglobin/iron is no longer sequestered in the cell). Paramagnetic iron has a greater shortening effect on T1 relaxation times. Diamagnetic iron is an iron molecule with no unpaired electron in its outer orbit and has no exaggerated T1 or susceptibility effects.

5.1. Hyperacute

At the immediate hyperacute phase, (upon bleeding into the parenchyma) iron is still saturated with oxygen (diamagnetic) and cell membranes are intact. Hence, the hematoma produces slight hypointensity ('darker') or iso-intensity ('same') on T1 weighted images and iso- or slightly hyperintense ('brighter') on T2 weighted images. This makes it hard to distinguish a hematoma at the extreme initial stages; however, as hemoglobin gets deoxygenated rapidly toward the periphery of the lesion, it produces a T2 hypointensity at the periphery (a dark rim), which helps detection in the hyperacute phase.

5.2. Acute

Within hours of the bleeding event, hemoglobin is deoxygenated within intact cell membranes, from the periphery to the center of the lesion which is paramagnetic. This causes a Susceptibility effect, which is hypointensity ('darker') on T2. However, this structure of hemoglobin does not allow any effect on T1 images, which show a hard to distinguish iso-('same') or slight hypo ('darker') lesion. At times, there is a peripheral rim of T1 hyperintensity due to early oxidation of hemoglobin into met-hemoglobin.

5.3. Subacute

This phase begins after several days with the onset hemoglobin degradation. Due to the lack of energy in the cells, the iron is oxidized into the ferric state, which produces met-hemoglobin. This structure of iron atoms causes a decrease in the T1 relaxation times which is captured as a marked hyperintensity ('brighter') on T1 weighted images. Since the red cell membranes are intact, Susceptibility effect is in play causing a hypo ('darker') appearance on T2 weighted images.

Later on in the subacute phase (over days to weeks), the red cell membranes are degraded; hence the susceptibility effect is lost. This results in a T2 lengthening, which is seen as a hyperintensity ('brighter') on T2 weighted images.

5.4. Chronic

Over the course of weeks to months, the resolution process results in protein (met-hemoglobin) breakdown, which reduces the signal hyperintensity on both T1 and T2 weighted images. The iron atoms released in this process are picked up by macrophages and converted to ferritin for reuse elsewhere. However, the scavenging capacity of the macrophages is often overwhelmed especially in larger hematomas, which results in locally deposited hemosiderin molecules usually at the periphery. The structure of iron in hemosiderin exerts only a Susceptibility effect which is a hypointense ('darker') rim on T2 weighted images. The center of the hematoma may resolve into a cavity, usually filled with cerebrospinal fluid with the corresponding signal characteristics ('darker' on T1 weighted imaging and 'brighter' on T2 weighted imaging) or may collapse and be visualized as a narrow slit.

While the pathological processes usually follow a sequence with corresponding sequential imaging changes, these processes are also highly variable and dependent on a large number of factors such as size, presence of rebleed, oxygen tension, other concurrent conditions etc. Hence several stages of the hematoma may appear simultaneously on imaging which increases the complexity of determining the time of bleed.

MR is also a tool in neuroimaging to distinguish between a primary bleed and a hemorrhagic transformation, since area of the bleed is usually lesser than area of the infarct, and MR provides imaging of both. The shape (rounder) and larger edema around the bleed is another pointer toward primary ICH. Hematomas do not follow vascular territories but infarcts do and the occlusion is often visible on MR angiography.

http://dx.doi.org/10.5772/67303

MR is also one of the best diagnostic tools for secondary causes of hemorrhage, such as vascular anomalies, tumors, and cerebral venous thrombosis (comparable to conventional angiography) and is the choice of modality for cavernomas. It has a high diagnostic yield for etiologies especially in young nonhypertensive patients with lobar bleeds.

5.5. MRI-sequences in ICH

MR protocols in stroke include T1, T2, T2* or GRE, fluid attenuated inversion recovery (FLAIR), contrast enhanced, diffusion weighted & perfusion weighted images, and MR angiography. Since the radiological appearance of the hematoma depends on both the hematoma and the MR signal characteristics, the latter can be varied to allow easier identification of hemorrhage. This is crucial as MRI shows minor and hard to appreciate changes in the hyperacute and early-acute phases of ICH. By increasing the magnetic field, the susceptibility effect is increased, allowing easier and more rapid diagnosis. Sequences available commonly in clinical practice include fast spin echo (FSE), which due to a weaker magnetic field has less sensitivity to susceptibility effects (responsible for much of the lesion imaging) and is hence suboptimal initially in ICH detection. Using sequences such as gradient recalled echo (GRE) and echo planar imaging (EPI) increases the sensitivity to susceptibility effect.

5.6. GRE

Gradient recalled echo sequences (or T2* weighted sequence) increases the hematoma detection in both acute and chronic stages. The strong Susceptibility effect results in extremely hypointense areas of hemorrhage on imaging (**Figure 3**).

T2* GRE MRI sequence has high sensitivity in detecting cerebral microbleeds, which appear as small punctate (dot-like) hypo-intense lesions widespread in bilateral cerebral cortical white matter , basal ganglia , thalami, cerebellum as well as brain stem and are histologically characterized by hemosiderin deposits with tissue damage.

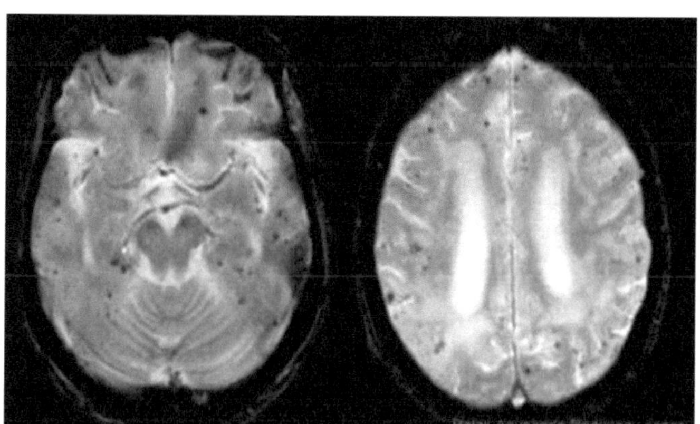

Figure 3. Gradient recalled echo. T2* GRE MRI sequence has high sensitivity in detecting cerebral microbleeds, which appear as small punctate (dot-like) hypointense lesions widespread in bilateral cerebral cortical white matter, basal ganglia, thalami, cerebellum, as well as brain stem and are histologically characterized by hemosiderin deposits with tissue damage.

An advantage of GRE is that it can exclusively identify hemosiderin deposits from old and asymptomatic hemorrhages often referred to as microbleeds. A large number of microbleeds point to an etiology such as amyloid angiopathy or recurrent hypertensive vasculopathy. Since 80% of the hemosiderin deposits persist through a lifetime, it provides a snapshot of the hemorrhages across the patient's life span. These microbleeds are used as predictors of future ICH and a marker for small vessel disease especially in the basal ganglia region. The disadvantage in this sequence is occasionally the lesion size, which is inaccurate due to artifacts causing signal loss at the boundary of the lesions. Sinuses present in the skull enhance this signal loss and may not allow accurate identification of hemorrhagic lesions behind them [5].

6. Catheter angiogram in ICH

Certain clinical and radiological findings necessitate a conventional catheter angiogram, such as atypical configuration or location, excessive edema, evidence of masses or no obvious cause of bleeding; all of which necessitate pinpointing a secondary cause. The diagnostic yield of a conventional angiogram is high especially in younger patients with no hypertension. Often times, the vascular anomaly reveals itself over the course of time (upon resolution) and hence a follow up angiogram is recommended even after a prior workup reveals no abnormality. However, significant disadvantages of conventional angiography that include extremely high (5× more than CTA) radiation, cost, invasiveness, patient cooperation, and clinical stability as well as transient and permanent neurological deficits preclude its widespread use, giving preference to CT and MR angiography but remain the gold standard for aneurysms and arteriovenous malformations.

7. Detecting the etiology of ICH

An important step in the management of patients with ICH is determining the etiology and taking measures to correct and prevent further and future episodes of ICH. While medical history and demographics may help pinpoint a cause for the ICH, neuroimaging has a large role to play in this sphere.

Neuroimaging can provide a clue to etiology of the ICH based on the **location** and **imaging characteristics** of the hemorrhage.

Each **location or area** of the brain is associated with a list of common differentials as to possible etiologies. Lobar hemorrhage (bleeding mainly into the cortex through the sub-cortical junction) is mainly superficial and as the name states, deep ICH refers to bleeding mainly in the deeper structures such as thalamus, putamen, and head of the caudate. Lobar hemorrhages are usually not related to hypertension but are caused by cerebral amyloid angiopathy (including in patients with hypertension) and are present in the white matter of the cerebrum and rarely in the cerebellum. Most deep or non-lobar ICHs are usually due to hypertension which is usually diagnosed based on the hemorrhage location. Hypertensive ruptures usually affect the smaller vessels such as lenticulostriate arteries, and perforating branches of the basilar artery, resulting in the characteristic sites of ICH. This lobar vs. deep structure based diagnosis does not hold true in patients less than 45 years of age where secondary causes such as vascular malformation, underlying tumor, vasoconstriction by sympathetic drugs are the usual culprits [7].

Hemorrhage in the brainstem (usually the pons) is usually associated with hypertension, vascular malformations (arteriovenous and cavernous).

Cerebellar hemorrhage is associated with hypertension, arteriovenous malformations, and the use of anticoagulants such as warfarin, with amyloid angiopathy being extremely rare.

Intraventricular hemorrhage (primarily intraventricular without involvement of the brain parenchyma) is associated with hypertension, aneurysm of the anterior communicating artery, vascular malformations, coagulopathy, and intraventricular tumors.

Hemorrhage at multiple sites is usually indicative of coagulation disorders, vasculitis, hypertension, tumors, and infarction.

Rupture of a saccular aneurysm may involve the parenchyma as well as the subarachnoid space, due to the pressure of the blood as it ruptures and its location (medial frontal lobe due to anterior cerebral or communicating artery aneurysm). Presence of ICH near the subarachnoid space near the base of the skull should prompt vascular imaging studies to rule out saccular aneurysms.

Common causes of ICH have distinctive **imaging characteristics** that point toward their diagnosis. The presence of multiple lobar microhemorrhages of differing ages, typically sparing the basal ganglia is a strong and specific indicator of cerebral amyloid angiopathy in the elderly which has been used in the clinical diagnostic criteria. The ICH in amyloid angiopathy often ruptures into the subarachnoid space but less commonly into the ventricles.

Arteriovenous malformations can often be suspected on conventional MRI and CT (T2 and MR and CT angiography) sequences by detecting dilated vessels to and from the malformation and at times patchy enhancement but are often times undetectable or silent. The presence of "popcorn" appearance of lesions on T2 weighted images suggests the presence of multiple small bleeds occurring at different time points in the same lesion such as a cavernous malformation. Presence of multiple micro- or larger bleeds on GRE sequence is also suggestive of a vascular anomaly as an etiology. The diagnosis of these malformations generally requires conventional angiography for confirmation.

Hemorrhagic transformation of an infarct is suggested by the surrounding cytotoxic edema which follows the arterial boundaries unless the hemorrhage is severe and early enough to blur the infarct visualization (**Figure 4**).

Hemorrhagic transformation of an ischemic infarct evident on MRI. A: T2 GRE showing areas of hypo-intensity (yellow arrowhead) corresponding to hemorrhage. B: FLAIR sequence showing the edema associated with bleed (red arrowhead).

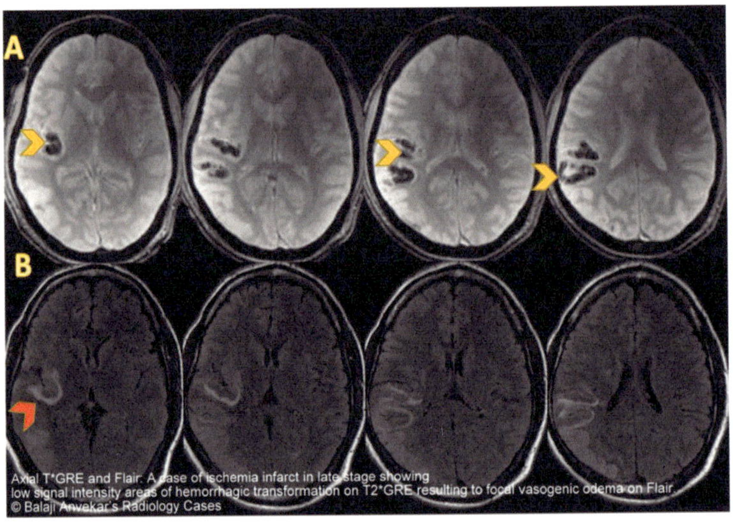

Figure 4. Hemorrhagic transformation. Hemorrhagic transformation of an ischemic infarct evident on MRI. A: T2 GRE showing areas of hypointensity (yellow arrowheads) corresponding to hemorrhage. B: FLAIR sequence showing the edema associated with bleed (red arrowhead).

Several neoplasms in the brain have a known propensity to bleed such as glioblastoma multiforme, and metastases of melanoma, lung cancer, renal cell cancer, etc. The imaging characteristics are variable due to the presence of often multiple hemorrhages at different time points and concurrent necrosis and cysts. Due to the low oxygen partial pressure in the tumor, MR signal changes are usually delayed. The location may be atypical for other common causes. The vasogenic edema present around a tumor is usually extensive and lasts longer as compared to primary ICH. Giving contrast almost always shows robust enhancement. A large hemorrhage may obscure the underlying lesion which may be visible on repeat imaging after its resolution [5].

8. Detecting complications of ICH

Complications of ICH include hematoma expansion, perilesional edema with increased intracranial pressure, and intraventricular extension of hemorrhage with hydrocephalus, seizures, venous thrombosis, hyperglycemia, autonomic fluctuations, and infections. Close monitoring is required for the prevention of these complications, and/or early detection and management, to reduce negative outcomes, the most emergent being mass effect resulting in herniation (**Figure 5**).

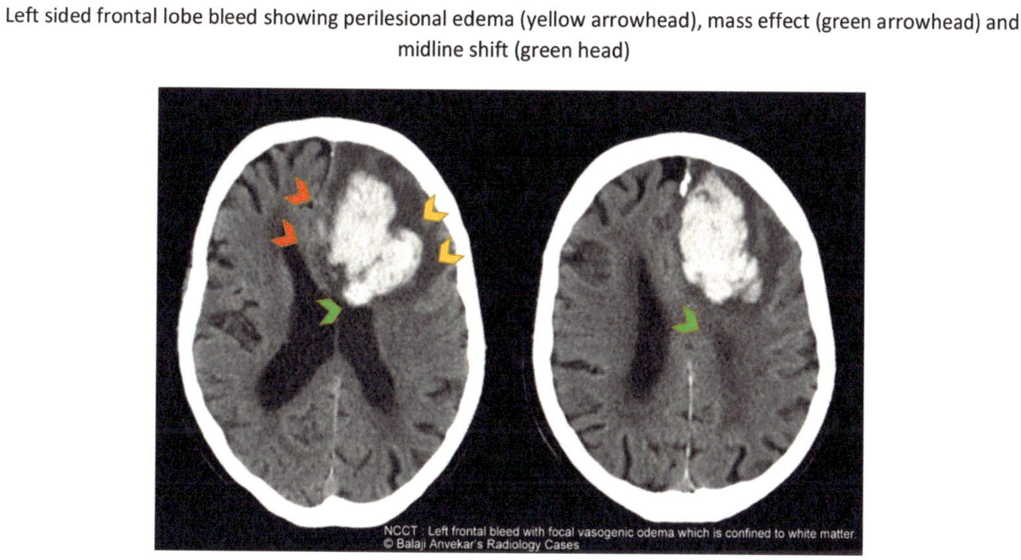

Figure 5. Detecting complications. Left sided frontal lobe bleed showing perilesional edema (yellow arrowheads), mass effect (green arrowheads) and midline shift (green arrowheads).

Since vasospasm in SAH (and uncommonly in ICH with intraventricular extension) is a known risk factor from day 3 to day 12, transcranial Doppler is used prophylactically for its screening, with variable results as compared to conventional angiography [8]. CTA is also used for this purpose, with high sensitivity and specificity for severe spasms and in proximal vessels but reduced accuracy for distal vessels and mild spasms [9]. Irrespective of vasospasm, neuroimaging for ischemia can be performed using CT or MR perfusion studies or diffusion weighted MRI. CT perfusion studies show great prediction of vasospasm as compared to conventional angiogram [10] and studies exploring blood brain barrier permeability to guide future treatments using CTP are underway [11].

Size of the ventricles measured on CT and MR is variable and is not accurate to diagnose hydrocephalus, although serial changes in size on the same patient is more relevant toward detection. Periventricular edema seen with transependymal flow is a marker of hydrocephalus, better seen on MR than CT [12].

9. Sequences in practice

9.1. Prognostication

The initial volume of the hematoma assessed by various methods on neuroimaging, commonly the ABC/2 method, the presence of intraventricular blood, as well as the expansion of the hematoma indicated by the 'spot sign' are independent markers for clinical outcomes and mortality [2, 13, 14] (**Table 3, Figure 6**).

	Advantage	Disadvantages
CT scan		
Availability	Faster, cheaper, widely available.	
Contraindication	Can be performed in patients with contraindications to MRI.	Contrast allergy and impaired renal function (for contrast administration).
Side effects		High dose of radiation, contrast associated side effects: allergy, nephropathy and variable effects on blood brain barrier permeability and cytotoxic edema.
Imaging: detection of blood	Due to the differential attenuation of blood (proportional to the protein concentration in blood) vs. gray and white matter, blood in the parenchyma is detected immediately.	Since imaging is based on protein concentration; detection difficult anemic patients (hemoglobin <10 g/dl). Patients with higher hematocrit such as infants will show abnormal density in vessels.
Imaging: location		Bleeds in brainstem can be obscured by artifact. Flattened and thin blood collections (such as subarachnoid) are hard to visualize.
Imaging characteristics		Differential diagnosis of hemorrhagic tumor vs. infarct is difficult. Ring enhancement of the blood seen 1–6 weeks after the bleed is hard to differentiate from other ring enhancing lesions. Age estimation of hematoma is not as accurate.
Immediate detection of hemorrhage	Gold standard noncontrast CT.	
Detecting perfusion deficits	CT angiography and CT perfusion imaging can be used to detect ischemia, and vasospasm.	
Detecting hemorrhagic conversion of infarcts	Bleeding detected immediately.	
Detecting chronic micro-bleeds		Not ideal.
Detecting etiology	CTA performed less than 96 h from onset are highly sensitive and specific for vascular malformations.	
MRI		
Availability		Not as fast/cheap or widely available.
Contraindication		Several; including pacemakers, metallic implants and claustrophobia.
Side effects	No radiation.	Nephrogenic systemic fibrosis associated with gadolinium.
Imaging: detection of blood	MRI is sensitive to flow abnormalities in vessels and is ideal for detecting vascular malformations.	Immediate bleeding is isointense but due to rapid deoxygenation of hemoglobin at periphery, shows hypointense periphery ion T2 and GRE.

	Advantage	Disadvantages
Imaging: location	Accurate at detecting exact location of hemorrhage.	
Imaging characteristics	Age estimation of hematoma is possible due to the differential magnetic properties of the different oxidation states of iron.	
Immediate detection of hemorrhage	MRI is sensitive if not more than CT in detecting acute ICH as per the HEME (Hemorrhage and Early MRI Evaluation) Study.	Gold standard remains noncontrast CT.
Detecting perfusion deficits	DWI/PWI mismatch.	
Detecting hemorrhagic conversion of infarcts	Ideal for distinguishing primary ICH vs. hemorrhagic conversion and shows the details of ischemic area.	
Detecting chronic micro-bleeds	More accurate than CT (GRE sequence). Lifetime history of hemorrhages is possible.	
Detecting etiology	Most sensitive and specific for detecting secondary causes such as vascular anomalies, venous thrombosis.	

*GRE = gradient recalled echo, CTA = computed tomography angiography, DWI = diffusion weighted imaging, PWI = perfusion weighted imaging.

Table 3. Advantages and disadvantages of CT and MRI in ICH imaging.

The risk of hemorrhage after ischemic lesions, notably after TPA administration, can be predicted by increased diffusion weighted imaging (DWI) lesion volumes, lower apparent diffusion coefficients, as well as decreased cerebral blood volume estimated using perfusion weighted imaging, the combination of the latter with DWI allowing one to identify infarcts with the colloquially termed 'malignant profile' for post thrombolytics bleeds. However, due to the time constraint of TPA administration which may not permit the above tools, CT perfusion imaging is being studied to predict similar hemorrhagic risk post thrombolysis based on the blood brain barrier permeability [15].

Using neuroimaging to correlate risk factors and measurable tissue states could allow greater precision in risk assessment. This could be utilized to predict the occurrence of ICH in patients of cerebral amyloid angiopathy (CAA) using PET and diffusion tensor imaging (DTI) [15].

While CT and MR provide the structural evidence of changes post ICH, aspects of brain function such as metabolism and absorption available through functional brain imaging may provide more granular details necessary to study the extent of injury and repair/recovery and may provide a new avenue to detect tissue at risk of hemorrhage.

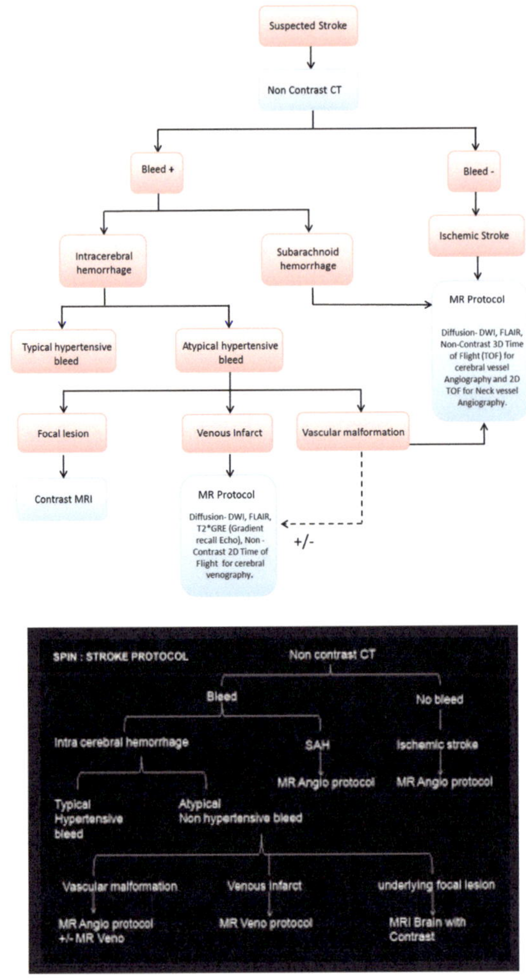

Figure 6. Sequencing protocol. Adapted with permission from Neuroradiologycases.com by Dr. Anvekar B. (Neuroradiology unit, S P Institute of Neurosciences, Solapur, India).

DTI can be used to detect disturbances to the integrity and fiber counts of white matter tract, often damaged in ICH. Reduced fractional anisotropy or fiber counts may suggest worsened outcomes [15]. DTI can be used to predict motor recovery, as patients with preserved tracts on DTI at the time of lesion have shown greater recovery than their counterparts with compromised tracts [16] with similar studies being carried out using fractional anisotropy. A significant finding being that fractional anisotropy ratio did not correlate to size of the bleed but did correlate with recovery [17], which could serve as an important tool for the prediction of recovery post ICH. The predictive value of these studies has shown to be higher when carried out subacutely (2 weeks) rather than acutely (3 days) after the bleed which may be accounted for by the resolution of acute injury and inflammation and onset of repair and compensation [18].

Functional MRI (fMRI) is being evaluated as a means to evaluate the extent of injury and functional deficit post ICH based on functional connectivity rather than just a structural basis, with fMRI possibly evaluating the activity between physical and functional connections. Studies have pointed to the subcortical origin of redistribution of functional connection when cortical motor tracts are damaged [19]. This expands the possibilities to create a precise model to predict recovery post ICH.

10. Newer imaging techniques

Several newer imaging technologies such as CT and MR perfusion, positron emission tomography (PET), single photon emission computed tomography (SPECT) are used to study tissue injury such as perfusion deficits around the hematoma. Studies using PET have shown that this hypoperfusion does not result in hypoxia and ischemia, thus is not frankly ischemic in origin but likely to be due to secondary metabolic failure [20]. Diffusion tensor imaging (DTI), used to visualize white matter tracts is being used and studied for prognostication on motor recovery by assessing the integrity of major motor pathways such as the corticospinal tract [16, 21]. Newer technological advances in CT include dynamic angiography (4-dimensional CT angiography) which allows a detailed and comprehensive visualization of the intra and extra cranial vasculature and perfusion using a 320-row setup [22]. Magnetic induction tomography is being studied to measure tissue conductivity noninvasively, allowing identification of pathological changes and identification of extremely minute blood volumes [23]. Further exploration is underway to expand the mandate of neuroimaging, allowing image guided therapy at specific time points, using imaging biomarkers to assess edema, inflammation, and excitotoxicity.

11. Conclusion

Neuroimaging is a constantly evolving field to optimize the management, and prognostication after intracerebral hemorrhage and to advance research efforts. There are several choices available for neuroimaging in patients of ICH and familiarizing oneself with the techniques, indications, and disadvantages of each method allows the development of a rational imaging plan. Several advances have been made in the image sequencing protocols to optimize detecting, diagnosing, and selecting candidates for intervention and other therapies. Advances in this field such as diffusion tensor imaging and functional MRI are being studied for their impact in understanding the extent of injury and possible recovery mechanisms possibly allowing precise prognostication for patients. The mandate of neuroimaging is ever expanding with the ultimate goal of discovering tools that remain sensitive, specific, safe, rapid, and widely available, which allows optimized prognosis, prevention, and management for the best possible patient outcomes.

Author details

Shazia Mirza[1*] and Sankalp Gokhale[2]

*Address all correspondence to: shazia.mirza@utsouthwestern.edu

1 UT Southwestern Medical Center, Dallas, USA

2 Banner University Medical Center, University of Arizona College of Medicine, Tucson, USA

References

[1] Rincon, F. and Mayer, S.A., The epidemiology of intracerebral hemorrhage in the United States from 1979 to 2008. Neurocrit Care, 2013. **19**(1): pp. 95-102.

[2] Macellari, F., et al., Neuroimaging in intracerebral hemorrhage. Stroke, 2014. **45**(3): pp. 903-8.

[3] Morgenstern, L.B., et al., Guidelines for the management of spontaneous intracerebral hemorrhage: A guideline for healthcare professionals from the American Heart Association/American Stroke Association. Stroke, 2010. **41**(9): pp. 2108-29.

[4] Siddiqui, F.M., Bekker, S.V., and Qureshi, A.I., Neuroimaging of hemorrhage and vascular defects. Neurotherapeutics, 2011. **8**(1): pp. 28-38.

[5] Smith, E.E., Rosand, J., and Greenberg, S.M., Imaging of hemorrhagic stroke. Magn Reson Imaging Clin N Am, 2006. **14**(2): pp. 127-40, v.

[6] Pedraza, S., et al., Reliability of the ABC/2 method in determining acute infarct volume. J Neuroimaging, 2012. **22**(2): pp. 155-9.

[7] Zhu, X.L., Chan, M.S., and Poon, W.S., Spontaneous intracranial hemorrhage: which patients need diagnostic cerebral angiography? A prospective study of 206 cases and review of the literature. Stroke, 1997. **28**(7): pp. 1406-9.

[8] Lysakowski, C., et al., Transcranial Doppler versus angiography in patients with vasospasm due to a ruptured cerebral aneurysm: A systematic review. Stroke, 2001. **32**(10): pp. 2292-8.

[9] Greenberg, E.D., et al., Diagnostic accuracy of CT angiography and CT perfusion for cerebral vasospasm: A meta-analysis. AJNR Am J Neuroradiol, 2010. **31**(10): pp. 1853-60.

[10] Wintermark, M., et al., Visual grading system for vasospasm based on perfusion CT imaging: Comparisons with conventional angiography and quantitative perfusion CT. Cerebrovasc Dis, 2008. **26**(2): pp. 163-70.

[11] Kishore, S., et al., Perfusion-CT assessment of blood–brain barrier permeability in patients with aneurysmal subarachnoid hemorrhage. J Neuroradiol, 2012. **39**(5): pp. 317-25.

[12] Bradley, W.G., Jr., Diagnostic tools in hydrocephalus. Neurosurg Clin N Am, 2001. **12**(4): pp. 661-84, viii.

[13] Broderick, J.P., et al., Volume of intracerebral hemorrhage. A powerful and easy-to-use predictor of 30-day mortality. Stroke, 1993. **24**(7): pp. 987-93.

[14] Davis, S.M., et al., Hematoma growth is a determinant of mortality and poor outcome after intracerebral hemorrhage. Neurology, 2006. **66**(8): pp. 1175-81.

[15] McDowell, M.M., et al., The role of advanced neuroimaging in intracerebral hemorrhage. Neurosurg Focus, 2013. **34**(4): p. E2.

[16] Cho, S.H., et al., Motor outcome according to the integrity of the corticospinal tract determined by diffusion tensor tractography in the early stage of corona radiata infarct. Neurosci Lett, 2007. **426**(2): pp. 123-7.

[17] Yoshioka, H., et al., Diffusion tensor tractography predicts motor functional outcome in patients with spontaneous intracerebral hemorrhage. Neurosurgery, 2008. **62**(1): pp. 97-103; discussion 103.

[18] Wang, D.M., et al., Diffusion tensor imaging predicts long-term motor functional outcome in patients with acute supratentorial intracranial hemorrhage. Cerebrovasc Dis, 2012. **34**(3): pp. 199-205.

[19] Jang, S.H., et al., Demonstration of motor recovery process in a patient with intracerebral hemorrhage. NeuroRehabilitation, 2007. **22**(2): pp. 141-5.

[20] Kidwell, C.S. and Wintermark, M., Imaging of intracranial haemorrhage. Lancet Neurol, 2008. **7**(3): pp. 256-67.

[21] Hosomi, A., et al., Assessment of arcuate fasciculus with diffusion-tensor tractography may predict the prognosis of aphasia in patients with left middle cerebral artery infarcts. Neuroradiology, 2009. **51**(9): pp. 549-55.

[22] Siebert, E., et al., Neuroimaging by 320-row CT: Is there a diagnostic benefit or is it just another scanner? A retrospective evaluation of 60 consecutive acute neurological patients. Neurol Sci, 2010. **31**(5): pp. 585-93.

[23] Chen, Y., et al., Imaging hemorrhagic stroke with magnetic induction tomography: Realistic simulation and evaluation. Physiol Meas, 2010. **31**(6): pp. 809-27.

Chapter 5

Intracerebral Hemorrhage: Issues in Rehabilitation

Ravi Dadlani and Amit Agrawal

Additional information is available at the end of the chapter

http://dx.doi.org/10.5772/intechopen.70586

Abstract

While the advancements in the management of the spontaneous intracerebral hemorrhage (SICH) have resulted an increase in survival, this has also resulted in the number of survivors with significant functional morbidity that require long-term care and rehabilitation services. SICH can lead to various impairments, and the deficits related to SICH may include impairment in motor and sensory functions, emotional labiality, language dysfunctions, perception deficits and cognitive dysfunctions. In the present chapter, we present an overview of the issues in rehabilitation which are faced by medical personnel's while managing the patients with SICH.

Keywords: intracerebral hemorrhage, physical impairment, disability, rehabilitation

1. Introduction

Spontaneous intracerebral hemorrhage (SICH) is characterized by nontraumatic bleeding into the brain parenchyma [1]. Further the term "primary spontaneous intracerebral hemorrhage" denotes a spontaneous hemorrhage into the brain parenchyma without any secondary cause (i.e., vascular abnormality, brain tumor, etc.) [2]. SICH accounts for approximately 10–20% of all stroke cases, carries a 30-day mortality of up to 50%, and causes significant and persistent disability in survivors [3–7]. Advances in the management of the SICH have resulted an increase in survival, particularly in cases of smaller lesions; however, larger SICH lesions remain a significant cause of morbidity and mortality globally [8, 9]. Literature suggests that in comparison with ischemic stroke, SICH causes more morbidity and mortality [10]. SICH can lead to various impairments including motor and cognitive deficits, sensorimotor impairment, impaired mobility, depression, swallowing dysfunctions, constipation and urinary incontinence [11]. The rehabilitation in SICH patients is targeted to facilitate the recovery process, avoid complications and optimize the functional outcomes acute as well as well as in post-acute recovery phase [11].

2. Overall management

The management of SICH can be divided into medical management, surgical management (when indicated) and rehabilitation both in acute as well as post-acute recovery phase [12]. The medical and surgical management intend to stabilize the general as well as the neurological condition of the patient and to prevent the secondary brain injury (either due to mass effect or presence of clotted blood in the brain parenchyma) [13–15]. In the acute phase, the major medical complications that can occur includes pneumonia (because of dysphagia and aspiration), aspiration, respiratory failure/distress, pulmonary embolism and sepsis [16, 17]. The most important step in the initial management, is the control of hypertension, which is the major risk factor that increases the risk of developing SICH by approximately four times [2].

3. Rehabilitation concepts

The deficits related to SICH are variable and may include impairment in motor and sensory functions, emotional labiality, language dysfunctions, perception deficits, and cognitive dysfunctions [18]. A number of factors decide the functional outcome as well as the treatment protocol for a given patient. While assessing a patient with SICH for rehabilitation, we need to identify whether the stroke has affected the dominant or nondominant side, whether the patient is having monoplegia, hemiplegia, or any other paralytic syndromes, are there any cognitive or speech disturbances (i.e., aphasia, dysphasia, dysarthria or fluency disorder), whether there is impairment of swallowing or if the patient is on tracheostomy. Additionally, this detailed evaluation should detect the presence of any pressure ulcers, their numbers and sites. Neuroplasticity is often regarded as a physiological basis for recovery after brain insults [19]. There is a dearth of reliable efficient post-stroke rehabilitative therapy implying a significant clinical need [20–22], and there is a significant "therapeutic window" that exists for the SICH patients to recover functionally [23].

4. Rehabilitation and recovery

In the case of hemorrhagic stroke, it has been documented in the literature that gait, limb motor and sensory function generally continue to recover until 3 months after onset; however, gait could improve up to 6 months from onset and it has been shown that upper limb recovery could persist up to an year [24]. This prolonged recovery is a witness to the beneficial outcome of rehabilitation during the subacute phase of recovery in stroke patients [25]. Neuronal plasticity is a subject of dedicated study today and is defined as the ability of the brain to recover functionally due to neuronal reorganization after a cerebral insult. It can usually occur actively following any cerebral insult, albeit for a limited time. It has been postulated that in acute phase and early stages of recovery following SICH delayed metabolic changes, continued neuronal damage and apoptosis in perihematomal tissue can continue to cause more active inflammatory damage, which is mediated by cellular and noncellular components, leading to more widespread consequences [26–30]. Thus, in comparison with an equivalent-sized ischemic infarct, in patients with SICH, an intraparenchymal blood leads to an increased inflammation and a greater cell death [26, 31]. There is growing evidence that recovery in functions is better in patients with SICH than in patients with ischemic strokes [6, 32–42]. The recovery process starts in the acute phase and can continue for months in the recovery phase [38, 43, 44].

5. Right versus left hemisphere stroke

There is a conflicting evidence whether which hemisphere stroke corroborates with a better outcome [45–47]. The controversy stems from various factors including the varied outcome scales used, measurement domain, presence of hemineglect and the timing of evaluation; for example, in considering vocational rehabilitation, patients with the right hemisphere stroke appear to have a better outcome [48]. The left hemisphere controls speech and language function along with the right half of the body. Strokes in this half of the brain demonstrate a right hemiplegia and aphasia [49]. Preservation of language function is considered one of the primary reasons for a higher percentage of right afflicted people returning to work; however, this cohort of patients are usually the one who most frequently develop social shortcomings in contrast to the left-sided stroke patients [50]. Further studies with exclusion of hemineglect patients may help to exemplify the difference in the disabilities between left and right hemisphere stroke patients [51].

6. Impaired motor function

Restoration of the motor function and mobility is one of the most important components of stroke rehabilitation [52]. Although most stroke patients regain walking independence, many have continuing problems with mobility due to impaired balance, motor weakness, and decreased walking velocity [18]. Impaired motor functions can be due to paralysis or paresis of the muscles (depending on the site of the lesion), which results from the damage to the brain parenchyma (motor cortex or descending/ascending pathways in the internal capsule and corona radiata), resulting in abnormal regulation of spinal motoneurons, alterations in postural and stretch reflexes and loss of voluntary movements [18, 53–56]. If the lesions involve the internal capsule, thalamus, periventricular white matter, and/or premotor cortex, the recovery of the upper limb motor functions is poorer [25, 57]. Regarding the functions in the lower limbs, in a study, it was shown that approximately 51% of subjects were without walking function at the time of admission to the rehabilitation unit and 12% of the subjects needed assistance during ambulation [58]. One of these patients was subjected to rehabilitation protocol, and the number of subjects with no walking function was reduced to 18% [58].

7. Sensory dysfunctions

Stroke survivors may have sensory impairment that may be either central or peripheral. The latter includes loss of primary sensory modalities such as hypoesthesia/paresthesia, proprioception and position sense loss or loss of pain and temperature sensations, or they may have more complex sensory impairments such as agraphesthesia and astereognosis, which are impairments of the central sensory mechanisms [49]. These contribute to requiring additional assistance for these patients to relearn cognitive and motor skills. The processing of sensory modalities begins with reception which is the registration of the pure sensations and stimuli received from the various sensory organs such as eyes, ears, nose, tongue, skin, joints and the internal organs. These received sensations are then rerouted to the corresponding primary sensory cortices. The interpretation of these received stimuli is called perception. Perception is a higher cortical function of the brain involving various regions and is more complex than reception [49].

8. Cognitive dysfunction

Among all the factors portending a negative outcome, cognitive dysfunction has been described as the most potent [59, 60]. It has been suggested in recent studies that cognitive impairment and dementia may be reduced by satisfactory control of hypertension and by using drugs such as acetylcholinesterase inhibitors commonly used in Alzheimer's disease (donepezil, galantamine, rivastigmine) [61, 62]. A step forward in the pharmaceutical approach to post-stroke cognitive impairment, mainly related to language function, fluency and repetition, has been a randomized, placebo-controlled, double-blind study with levodopa which reported positive results [63].

9. Sphincter dysfunction

Usually, transient up to 20% of patients report persistence of urinary incontinence at discharge from rehabilitation [64, 65]. The commonest bladder dysfunction is the uninhibited bladder usually resolving with timed voiding training. Anticholinergic drugs such as tolterodine or oxybutynin may be indicated to relax the bladder. Sphincter recovery parallels and accompanies other functional recovery. Bladder unawareness in addition to lower limb weakness and cognitive impairment is a poor prognostic factor. Significant cognitive impairment may remain a lifelong disability [49]. Dual incontinence involving both bladder and bowel is much common than an isolated incontinence [65].

10. Other impairments and disabilities sequel to stroke

Many stroke survivors require tracheostomy, some permanently. This does increase the risk of pulmonary aspiration since laryngeal elevation during deglutition is impaired. Careful selection of the texture of food and scrupulous monitoring during swallowing are essential to prevent aspiration in these patients [49]. Post-stroke depression is notable and has been postulated to be the main reason for suicide in these patients [66]. Morbidity in many clinical scenarios is considered a worse outcome than death, especially in neurological disorders in which the patient may be "alive but dependent" [67].

11. Role of dedicated rehabilitation services

Exercise, in general, has been shown to impart several favorable effects in neural recovery [68, 69]. Rehabilitation of stroke patients is increasingly demanding as far as the resources are considered. In general, most rehabilitation units have inadequate resources making the selection process an imperative component of the assessment [37]. Stroke care units that incorporate rehabilitation services generally claim better clinical outcomes in comparison to other models of stroke care units [70]. A decreased incidence of mortality, morbidity and dependency have been reported in stroke patients who undergo therapeutic training in an inpatient unit than those who receive general rehabilitation in a nondedicated unit [71]. Medically stable neurological patients need to be placed in the best possible unit for which several deliberations need to be considered [11]. On termination of a course of inpatient rehabilitation, further therapy may be instituted on an outpatient basis or an extended functional training at home may be considered [11].

12. Conclusion

The overall outcome of the SICH patients depends on access to acute care facilities, availability and affordability of post-acute care and rehabilitation services. The provision of stroke rehabilitation services has received considerable attention in recent years. There is a large amount of literature that support the rehabilitation of acute and subacute phase of SICH that has potential for improvement in the functional outcome of these patients. However, more studies are needed to further define and compare different methods for rehabilitation in patients with SICH.

Author details

Ravi Dadlani[1]* and Amit Agrawal[2]

*Address all correspondence to: ravi.dadlani@gmail.com

1 Department of Neurosurgery, Apollo Specialty Hospitals, Nellore, Andhra Pradesh, India

2 Department of Neurosurgery, Narayana Medical College Hospital, Chinthareddypalem, Nellore, Andhra Pradesh, India

References

[1] Caplan LR. Intracerebral haemorrhage. The Lancet. 1992;**339**:656

[2] Qureshi AI, Tuhrim S, Broderick JP, Batjer HH, Hondo H, Hanley DF. Spontaneous intracerebral hemorrhage. New England Journal of Medicine. 2001;**344**:1450-1460

[3] Sacco S, Marini C, Toni D, Olivieri L, Carolei A. Incidence and 10-year survival of intracerebral hemorrhage in a population-based registry. Stroke. 2009;**40**:394-399

[4] Vermeer SE, Algra A, Franke CL, Koudstaal PJ, Rinkel GJE. Long-term prognosis after recovery from primary intracerebral hemorrhage. Neurology. 2002;**59**:205-209

[5] Fogelholm R, Murros K, Rissanen A, Avikainen S. Long term survival after primary intracerebral haemorrhage: A retrospective population based study. Journal of Neurology, Neurosurgery & Psychiatry. 2005;**76**:1534-1538

[6] Fogelholm R, Nuutila M, Vuorela AL. Primary intracerebral haemorrhage in the Jyväskylä region, central Finland, 1985-89: Incidence, case fatality rate, and functional outcome. Journal of Neurology, Neurosurgery & Psychiatry. 1992;**55**:546-552

[7] Broderick J, Brott T, Tomsick T, Leach A. Lobar hemorrhage in the elderly. The undiminishing importance of hypertension. Stroke. 1993;**24**:49-51

[8] Zahuranec DB, Gonzales NR, Brown DL, et al. Presentation of intracerebral haemorrhage in a community. Journal of Neurology, Neurosurgery & Psychiatry. 2006;**77**:340-344

[9] Morgenstern LB, Hemphill JC, Anderson C, et al. Guidelines for the management of spontaneous intracerebral hemorrhage. Stroke. 2010;**41**:2108-2129

[10] Hårdemark HG, Wesslén N, Persson L. Influence of clinical factors, CT findings and early management on outcome in supratentorial intracerebral hemorrhage. Cerebrovascular Diseases. 1999;**9**:10-21

[11] Saulle MF, Schambra HM. Recovery and Rehabilitation after Intracerebral Hemorrhage. Seminars in Neurology. 2016;**36**:306-312

[12] Moon J-S, Janjua N, Ahmed S, et al. Prehospital neurologic deterioration in patients with intracerebral hemorrhage. Critical Care Medicine. 2008;**36**:172-175

[13] Diringer MN, Edwards DF. Admission to a neurologic/neurosurgical intensive care unit is associated with reduced mortality rate after intracerebral hemorrhage. Critical Care Medicine. 2001;**29**:635-640

[14] Hemphill JC, Greenberg SM, Anderson CS, et al. Guidelines for the management of spontaneous intracerebral hemorrhage: A guideline for healthcare professionals from the American Heart Association/American Stroke Association. Stroke. 2015;**46**:2032-2060

[15] Alberts MJ, Latchaw RE, Selman WR, et al. Recommendations for comprehensive stroke centers: A consensus statement from the brain attack coalition. Stroke. 2005;**36**:1597-1616

[16] Lyden PD, Shuaib A, Lees KR, et al. Safety and tolerability of NXY-059 for acute intracerebral hemorrhage. Stroke. 2007;**38**:2262-2269

[17] Takahata H, Tsutsumi K, Baba H, Nagata I, Yonekura M. Early intervention to promote oral feeding in patients with intracerebral hemorrhage: A retrospective cohort study. BMC Neurology. 2011;**11**:6

[18] Peurala SH. Rehabilitation of Gait in Chronic Stroke Patients: University of Kuopio, 2005.

[19] Auriat AM, Wowk S, Colbourne F. Rehabilitation after intracerebral hemorrhage in rats improves recovery with enhanced dendritic complexity but no effect on cell proliferation. Behavioural Brain Research. 2010;**214**:42-47

[20] Hays SA, Rennaker RL, Kilgard MP. Targeting plasticity with vagus nerve stimulation to treat neurological disease. Progress in Brain Research. 2013;**207**:275

[21] Furmaga H, Carreno FR, Frazer A. Vagal nerve stimulation rapidly activates brain-derived neurotrophic factor receptor TrkB in rat brain. PLoS One. 2012;**7**:e34844

[22] Follesa P, Biggio F, Gorini G, et al. Vagus nerve stimulation increases norepinephrine concentration and the gene expression of BDNF and bFGF in the rat brain. Brain Research. 2007;**1179**:28-34

[23] Yang Y-R, Wang R-Y, Wang PS-G. Early and late treadmill training after focal brain ischemia in rats. Neuroscience Letters. 2003;**339**:91-94

[24] Rand D, Eng JJ. Predicting daily use of the affected upper extremity 1 year after stroke. Journal of Stroke and Cerebrovascular Diseases. 2015;**24**:274-283

[25] Lee KB, Kim JS, Hong BY, Kim YD, Hwang BY, Lim SH. The motor recovery related with brain lesion in patients with intracranial hemorrhage. Behavioural Neurology. 2015;**2015**:

[26] Xue M, Del Bigio MR. Intracerebral injection of autologous whole blood in rats: Time course of inflammation and cell death. Neuroscience Letters. 2000;**283**:230-232

[27] Gong C, Hoff JT, Keep RF. Acute inflammatory reaction following experimental intracerebral hemorrhage in rat. Brain Research. 2000;**871**:57-65

[28] Keep RF, Hua Y, Xi G. Intracerebral haemorrhage: Mechanisms of injury and therapeutic targets. The Lancet Neurology. 2012;**11**:720-731

[29] Donovan FM, Pike CJ, Cotman CW, Cunningham DD. Thrombin induces apoptosis in cultured neurons and astrocytes via a pathway requiring tyrosine kinase and RhoA activities. Journal of Neuroscience. 1997;**17**:5316-5326

[30] Carmichael ST, Vespa PM, Saver JL, et al. Genomic profiles of damage and protection in human intracerebral hemorrhage. Journal of Cerebral Blood Flow & Metabolism. 2008;**28**:1860-1875

[31] Xue M, Del Bigio MR. Intracortical hemorrhage injury in rats: Relationship between blood fractions and brain cell death. Stroke. 2000;**31**:1721-1727

[32] Daverat P, Castel JP, Dartigues JF, Orgogozo JM. Death and functional outcome after spontaneous intracerebral hemorrhage. A prospective study of 166 cases using multivariate analysis. Stroke. 1991;**22**:1-6

[33] Barber M, Roditi G, Stott DJ, Langhorne P. Poor outcome in primary intracerebral haemorrhage: Results of a matched comparison. Postgraduate Medical Journal. 2004;**80**:89-92

[34] Jørgensen HS, Nakayama H, Raaschou HO, Olsen TS. Intracerebral hemorrhage versus infarction: Stroke severity, risk factors, and prognosis. Annals of Neurology. 1995;**38**:45-50

[35] Lipson DM, Sangha H, Foley NC, Bhogal S, Pohani G, Teasell RW. Recovery from stroke: Differences between subtypes. International Journal of Rehabilitation Research. 2005;**28**:303-308

[36] Kelly PJ, Furie KL, Shafqat S, Rallis N, Chang Y, Stein J. Functional recovery following rehabilitation after hemorrhagic ischemic stroke. Archives of Physical Medicine and Rehabilitation. 2003;**84**:968-972

[37] Katrak PH, Black D, Peeva V. Do stroke patients with intracerebral hemorrhage have a better functional outcome than patients with cerebral infarction? PM&R. 2009;**1**:427-433

[38] Schepers VPM, Ketelaar M, Visser-Meily AJM, de Groot V, Twisk JWR, Lindeman E. Functional recovery differs between ischaemic and haemorrhagic stroke patients. Journal of Rehabilitation Medicine. 2008;**40**:487-489.

[39] Paolucci S, Antonucci G, Grasso MG, et al. Functional outcome of ischemic and hemorrhagic stroke patients after inpatient rehabilitation. Stroke. 2003;**34**:2861-2865

[40] Mestriner RG, Miguel PM, Bagatini PB, et al. Behavior outcome after ischemic and hemorrhagic stroke, with similar brain damage, in rats. Behavioural Brain Research. 2013;**244**:82-89

[41] Chae J, Zorowitz RD, Johnston MV. Functional outcome of hemorrhagic and nonhemorrhagic stroke patients after in-patient rehabilitation. American Journal of Physical Medicine & Rehabilitation. 1996;**75**:177-182

[42] Ween JE, Alexander MP, D'Esposito M, Roberts M. Factors predictive of stroke outcome in a rehabilitation setting. Neurology. 1996;**47**:388-392

[43] Hemphill JC, Farrant M, Neill TA. Prospective validation of the ICH score for 12-month functional outcome. Neurology. 2009;**73**:1088-1094

[44] Rost NS, Smith EE, Chang Y, et al. Prediction of functional outcome in patients with primary intracerebral hemorrhage: The FUNC score. Stroke. 2008;**39**:2304-2309

[45] Coughlan AK, Humphrey M. Presenile stroke: Long-term outcome for patients and their families. Rheumatology. 1982;**21**:115-122

[46] Goto A, Okuda S, Ito S, et al. Locomotion outcome in hemiplegic patients with middle cerebral artery infarction: The difference between right-and left-sided lesions. Journal of Stroke and Cerebrovascular Diseases. 2009;**18**:60-67

[47] Fink JN, Frampton CM, Lyden P, Lees KR. On behalf of the VI. Does hemispheric lateralization influence functional and cardiovascular outcomes after stroke?: An analysis of placebo-treated patients from prospective acute stroke trials. Stroke. 2008;**39**:3335-3340

[48] Howard G, Till JS, Toole JF, Matthews C, Truscott BL. Factors influencing return to work following cerebral infarction. Journal of the American Medical Association. 1985;**253**:226-232

[49] Kim C-T, Han J, Kim H. Pediatric stroke recovery: A descriptive analysis. Archives of Physical Medicine and Rehabilitation. 2009;**90**:657-662

[50] Mosch SC, Max JE, Tranel D. A matched lesion analysis of childhood versus adult-onset brain injury due to unilateral stroke: Another perspective on neural plasticity and recovery of social functioning. Cognitive and Behavioral Neurology. 2005;**18**:5-17

[51] Jehkonen M, Ahonen JP, Dastidar P, et al. Predictors of discharge to home during the first year after right hemisphere stroke. Acta Neurologica Scandinavica. 2001;**104**:136-141

[52] Jørgensen HS, Nakayama H, Raaschou HO, Olsen TS. Recovery of walking function in stroke patients: The Copenhagen stroke study. Archives of Physical Medicine and Rehabilitation. 1995;**76**:27-32

[53] Hardwick RM, Rottschy C, Miall RC, Eickhoff SB. A quantitative meta-analysis and review of motor learning in the human brain. NeuroImage. 2013;**67**:283-297

[54] Horovitz SG, Gallea C, Najee-ullah MA, Hallett M. Functional anatomy of writing with the dominant hand. PLoS One. 2013;**8**:e67931

[55] Planton S, Jucla M, Roux F-E, Démonet J-F. The "handwriting brain": A meta-analysis of neuroimaging studies of motor versus orthographic processes. Cortex. 2013;**49**:2772-2787

[56] Boudrias M-H, McPherson RL, Frost SB, Cheney PD. Output properties and organization of the forelimb representation of motor areas on the lateral aspect of the hemisphere in rhesus macaques. Cerebral Cortex. 2010;**20**:169-186

[57] de Nap Shelton F, Reding MJ. Effect of lesion location on upper limb motor recovery after stroke. Stroke 2001;**32**:107-112.

[58] Titianova EB, Pitkänen K, Pääkkönen A, Sivenius J, Tarkka IM. Gait characteristics and functional ambulation profile in patients with chronic unilateral stroke. American Journal of Physical Medicine & Rehabilitation. 2003;**82**:778-786

[59] Patel MD, Coshall C, Rudd AG, Wolfe CDA. Cognitive impairment after stroke: Clinical determinants and its associations with long-term stroke outcomes. Journal of the American Geriatrics Society. 2002;**50**:700-706

[60] Barker-Collo S, Feigin VL, Parag V, Lawes CMM, Senior H. Auckland stroke outcomes study part 2: Cognition and functional outcomes 5 years poststroke. Neurology. 2010;**75**:1608-1616

[61] Narasimhalu K, Effendy S, Sim CH, et al. A randomized controlled trial of rivastigmine in patients with cognitive impairment no dementia because of cerebrovascular disease. Acta Neurologica Scandinavica. 2010;**121**:217-224

[62] Rojas-Fernandez CH, Moorhouse P. Current concepts in vascular cognitive impairment and pharmacotherapeutic implications. Annals of Pharmacotherapy. 2009;**43**:1310-1323

[63] Seniów J, Litwin M, Litwin T, Leśniak M, Członkowska A. New approach to the rehabilitation of post-stroke focal cognitive syndrome: Effect of levodopa combined with speech and language therapy on functional recovery from aphasia. Journal of the Neurological Sciences. 2009;**283**:214-218

[64] Wilson DAN, Lowe D, Hoffman A, Rudd A, Wagg A. Urinary incontinence in stroke: Results from the UK National Sentinel Audits of stroke 1998-2004. Age and Ageing. 2008;**37**:542-546

[65] Kovindha A, Wattanapan P, Dejpratham P, Permsirivanich W, Kuptniratsaikul V. Prevalence of incontinence in patients after stroke during rehabilitation: A multi-centre study. Journal of Rehabilitation Medicine. 2009;**41**:489-491

[66] Brønnum-Hansen H, Davidsen M, Thorvaldsen P. Long-term survival and causes of death after stroke. Stroke. 2001;**32**:2131-2136

[67] Solomon NA, Glick HA, Russo CJ, Lee J, Schulman KA. Patient preferences for stroke outcomes. Stroke. 1994;**25**:1721-1725

[68] Ke Z, Yip SP, Li L, Zheng X-X, Tong K-Y. The effects of voluntary, involuntary, and forced exercises on brain-derived neurotrophic factor and motor function recovery: A rat brain ischemia model. PLoS One. 2011;**6**:e16643

[69] Pilc J. The effect of physical activity on the brain derived neurotrophic factor: From animal to human studies. Journal of Physiology and Pharmacology. 2010;**61**:533-541

[70] Chan DKY, Cordato D, O'Rourke F, et al. Comprehensive stroke units: A review of comparative evidence and experience. International Journal of Stroke. 2013;**8**:260-264

[71] Langhorne P, Duncan P. Does the organization of postacute stroke care really matter? Stroke. 2001;**32**:268-274